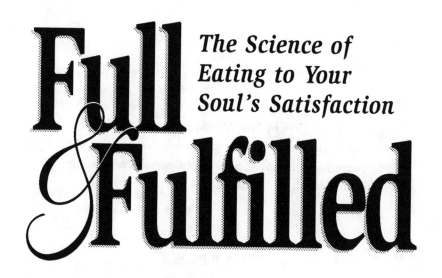

Full & Fulfilled

The Science of Eating to Your Soul's Satisfaction

Nan Allison, MS, RD
Carol Beck, MS

AB

A & B Books
2826 Azalea Place
Nashville, TN 37204

phone: 615/297-7888
fax: 615/297-9799
email: allisona@juno.com

Cover art: Carol Beck
Book design/production: PDQ Partners
Printed in the United States of America

ISBN 0-9659117-9-9

Acknowledgments

Thanks to all the reviewers who struggled through our first draft of this book: Dick Allison, Sara and Steve Lancaster, Mike O'Neil, Diane Sacks; a special note of thanks to Francis Bledsoe for doing a wonderful job of editing, as well. Thanks to all our professional writers, Lynn Bachleda, Amy Lynch, and Amy Lyles Wilson, who tried to help us put our ideas into words; to Mark Kaufman, who counseled us through every step of the way; to Keneth Langley, who formatted, reformatted, typed and retyped innumerable drafts with remarkable silence; to Lynn Bennett and F. Clark Williams, Jr. for their support and valuable insights; to all our close friends who have listened to us as we gave birth to this book—Elizabeth Crook, Peggy Evans, Genie James, Jan Liff, David Lloyd, Anne Miller, Jamie Morse, Peggy Schuyler, Diane Sacks; to Sarah Jane Freymann for being the first literary professional who believed in our manuscript; to Jenny Adams, Peggy Elam, Dawn Kimbrell, Ruth Ann Leach, Thom Rutledge, Bob Stepbach, Tom Ventress, Walberga Engel and other professional colleagues in the community who shared their wisdom with us; to all our *Intuitive Eating Newsletter* readers who encouraged us to actually write this book; to Jerry Campbell, Susan Austin-Crumpton, and Suzie Waters Benjamin for guiding us along our spiritual paths enough that we could write this book. Special thanks to Nan's family—parents, sisters and brothers-in-law, and to Carol's mom. And finally, to our clients, who have patiently taught us everything we know about intuitive eating.

Table of Contents

Section Three: Ending the Struggle

To our clients . . .
without you
this book would not be.

Introduction

Even with the best training from some of the most reputable nutrition schools in the nation, advanced degrees, and years of experience, we were still struggling to help our clients in their battles with food and weight.

Something was wrong.

We had been trying to find yet one more technique for better motivation—have clients visit more often, call more frequently, and learn more facts about food, nutrients, emotions and weight control. All these efforts were exhausting us and our clients; we got frustrated with them, and they with us. We talked with psychotherapists for perspectives on their clients' struggles with food. We experimented with the assumptions that

1   a lack of pleasure and satisfaction could play a role in this struggle (and tried mightily to have clients interject more pleasure and planned indulgences in their daily food routines); or

2   that some clients could be too busy to truly care for their bodies, so worked with them to find time for their bodies; or

3   that in this society, we have all been taught to discount, minimize, avoid, cover up, keep a stiff upper lip—anything but acknowledge our pain.

We recognized that all of these factors played a role in the reasons people eventually returned to eating in ways they always had, preventing them from making the changes they wanted to or thought they should make. But all of this information was not enough. Something was still missing.

Neither we nor our clients consciously realized the connection between where they were on their life paths and their behavior with food. Their best attempts to change food habits did not have lasting effects until they looked at the link between their bodies and their emotional and spiritual lives. The reason: experiencing the emotional and spiritual parts of us causes biochemical changes in our bodies which alter our desire for food. In addition, eating in a way which balances with the body's needs often gives people greater clarity in getting to know themselves as emotional and spiritual beings.

People can choose, then, to travel their paths by entering at either, or both, gateways—by working on food issues and moving on to the emotional/spiritual issues or vice versa. The important point is to recognize and understand that the two—cellular/biochemical and emotional/spiritual—are linked.

As you read the chapters in this book, you will begin to see the paradoxical relationship between your spiritual/emotional life, eating, and your physical body. How we eat and how we view our bodies are metaphors for handling life; our relationship with food says something about who we are and how we express our very being in the world. Not only are they metaphors, they are concrete, physical reflections of where we are on our life's path and can determine how we proceed.

So, don't stop dreaming about achieving peace with food. Most of us want that peace so desperately yet are stymied when using the strategies and options taught us. It is impossible to successfully use these strategies, however "right" they may be, without first knowing what feels good and right *for you*. Our bodies are filled with authentic clues about what is right for us but we have been taught to discount the very signals that free us to make the dream of peace with food a reality—to truly be full and fulfilled.

We finally realized that clients intuitively knew something that neither we nor they fully understood—what we now label the "intuitive eater" (body signals) within, and that the intuitive eater is the key to feeling both full and fulfilled. So we finally gave ourselves and our clients permission *not to know* the answers and trusted that our clients' bodies would eventually give them the clues they needed to begin to explore and discover their own inner wisdom.

This book is designed for you to do the same thing. Some clients choose to explore their food patterns and behavior, and in so doing, start to find the connection between their emotional/spiritual struggles and food intake. Others will find it more comfortable to explore their emotional/spiritual paths first. Either way, the biochemical balance in the body is altered, making it easier to then address the other. We wrote this book so that you, the reader, can begin to use the power that comes from listening to your intuitive eater; to begin trusting, interpreting, experimenting with, applying, and practicing using your intuitive eater. You have everything you need to feel both full *and* fulfilled. This book gives you both the permission and information you need to discover what's right for you.

What is Intuitive Eating?

Intuitive eating has certain characteristics:

It varies from person to person. Because our tastes, bodies, activities, emotions, and spiritual paths are different, what our bodies require in terms of nourishment also differs.

It is cyclical. Weekly, monthly, and annual cycles, even life cycles, change our body's need for, and responses to, food.

It is imperfect. Intuitive eating does not mean we'll always choose absolutely "healthy" or "pristine" foods. We won't always feel as if we've had a "perfect" balance.

It is rhythmic. We feel pleasantly full (but not stuffed) after a meal and pleasantly hungry (but not starving) before the next.

It includes a wide variety of foods. Cereals and grains, fruits and vegetables, dairy products, meats, beans, nuts, and even fats play a role in normal, intuitive eating. Again, the exact balance and variety of foods must be individualized.

It is free of obsession. It acknowledges that our compulsions are due to biochemical or emotional reasons and any over- or under-eating is a clue to begin looking further as an opportunity for learning.

It is nourishing to the body and spirit.

It feels good. Good food in the right amounts and at the right times excites the senses. It provides tactile and taste sensations as we eat, and a pleasurable "full" feeling afterward. When we finish a meal, we feel comforted and renewed—physically, emotionally, and even spiritually.

It is an essential component of self care. What better way to nurture ourselves than with the foods we need and enjoy in the amounts we require?

The Fight To Eat "Right"

If you are like most of us, you have struggled for a long time with food—or against it. Think about all the times you have turned down dessert (probably more occasions than you realize), and the times you didn't let yourself eat what you really wanted. In following a prescribed diet, you may fill yourself *full* of foods you actually hate while you come to despise foods you actually like, such as tuna, cottage cheese and Melba toast because you associate them with the "diet." You may eat combinations of foods which seem odd or unnatural to you. Maybe you measure or weigh every bite that goes into your mouth.

You work very hard to eat right—yet derive little or no lasting benefit. And, you may *continue to struggle*—your relationship with food does not become easier over time. Clearly, something is wrong with this picture! Work this hard ought to produce results. When it doesn't, the overall scheme of things needs to be revisited. This book helps you do just that. It helps you understand what is going on biochemically at the cellular level, how that is connected to what your mind is thinking, your heart is feeling and your soul is believing and how all these connections translate into the foods you are drawn to, the eating patterns you follow—your eating style. It's about how foods and your eating patterns affect your biochemistry in such a way that your heart and mind can open to your soul and grow at this deep level. This spiritual growth subsequently affects our drive for certain foods and ways of eating. So, eating not only keeps us connected to the physical world but can also allow us to grow as spiritual beings and listen to and care for our souls, not just our bodies.

Fighting the Wrong Battle

No wonder we lose the battle with food and weight over and over again. We were not born to fight it. In fact, so long as we continue to *fight* with food, we will never have all the energy we wish for, our scales will continue to show numbers that we don't want to see, and our reflections in the mirror will fail to please us. This is a battle we were never supposed to fight and are destined to lose. For we and food are meant to be natural allies—not enemies. We can go on fighting—many of us do for all our lives—but we can never win. We only grow weary.

Maybe you've been doing things that don't work because not only were you unaware of the impact of the spiritual/emotional/ biochemical connection in your life but also because the food plans and diets you've tried won't work (indeed, will *never* work) for you. Perhaps, along with millions of other people, you've been provided with rules about food that simply don't apply to you. We're assuming these rules and diet plans were based on each author's lifestyle and experience, and successfully might have helped *them* control their weight.

But, that does not mean their plans will work for you. For example, Oprah Winfrey found a nutritional system that worked for *her;* Richard Simmons has *his* own exercise and diet strategy; Susan Powter, author of the popular book, **Stop The Insanity**, found *her* way to a satisfying relationship with food. But, each of these programs was based on *individual* physical needs, personal tastes, schedules, and personalities.

Fortunately, there is another way. Here, in this book, *you* have a step-by-step guide to do exactly the same thing—only just for you, going even broader and deeper by incorporating your biochemical/emotional/spiritual connection.

The Journey of Discovery

This book is here to help you reclaim your intuitive eater within. It is here to help you give up your struggle with food. **Intuitive eating is a guided individual journey.** If you are looking for a list of do's and don'ts, or for a new set of battle plans, you will be disappointed. In fact, you will find very few case studies or client examples in this book. Those examples wouldn't be useful. Your relationship with food is yours alone. It's not like anybody else's. Intuitive eating is not a food plan, but an opportunity for you to explore your own reactions to, and experiences with, food. We encourage you to learn which foods please you, nourish and sustain you, and to learn about how your body and food interact.

Like any journey of discovery, intuitive eating takes time. Clients ask, *"How long does it take?"* Our answer: *"It takes as long as it takes."* Throughout the process, there will be times when a whole world of answers will open to you; other times, the insight gained will be more subtle. In fact, just by trying some of these experiments, things will change. You'll find there isn't one correct answer. Don't be surprised if you don't get the same results every time. What is real for you is based on the mode of consciousness that you bring to bear at each moment. Along the way, you will sometimes experience what feels like failure. But the effort is well worth the rewards. Each failure will provide insight to move you one step further along the path toward success. You will move to a place where you are:

♦ naturally, effortlessly, and comfortably eating foods you enjoy in moderate and healthy amounts

♦ eating when you are hungry, not starving

♦ stopping when you are full, not stuffed

♦ accepting, not panicking, when eating doesn't go just right.

Intuitive eating means feeling confidence and trust in yourself when it comes to food because you are learning to accept your body, emotions, and food, and the ways they work together.

Giving up old habits is not easy. Abandoning the struggle is—well—a struggle. As you explore intuitive eating you'll get to know food again. You will become sensitive to your body's needs and signals related to food, and its responses to your emotions and spiritual growth. You will re-examine old ideas and behaviors. You will take some risks.

Waking the Intuitive Self

The process of learning how to feel full and fulfilled will put you back in touch with your body so that you can "hear" its signals for certain kinds or amounts of food. In some ways, *finding the intuitive eater within is like waking a good friend from a lifetime slumber.* A gentle touch may be all you need. The knowledge that you carry inside you is like this sleeping friend—unconscious, but not deeply so, and waiting to be wakened.

Unfortunately, each of us also carries around vicious food prohibitions—notions imposed on us by others. We absorb these rules and regulations, which may not be right for us, in the effort to do the "right" thing or look the "right" way. Along with these rules are pieces of misinformation and misconceptions about how our bodies work. We also carry the feelings associated with them—shame, guilt, even fear. All those layers of misinformation and bad feelings must be recognized and peeled away before we can rediscover the memory of how good it feels to eat naturally and intuitively.

In this book, we will help you wake your intuition about food by combining:

⇒ facts about the way bodies work, how emotions influence bodies, and the role of food in the interaction between the two. This information will help you understand why you just haven't been able to do what it is you thought you were "supposed" to do with food. This knowledge will also give you "permission" to risk eating more intuitively.

⇒ activities to help you explore your inner knowledge, allowing you to recall old food-related experiences and create new ones. These discoveries will help you reorient your thinking about your body and the food you use to fuel it. They will also help you learn to make food choices with confidence.

Intuitive eating is a journey. This is its beginning. Expect the exhilaration and excitement of any journey, along with its discomforts. Anticipate moments of insight and surrender. The good news is that you need not make this trip alone. This text will be your guide. And your intuition, too, will journey with you. Now it is time to wake your intuitive eater from its slumber.

Section One:

Learning What's Missing

1

Discovering What's Right For You

> *"Plato argued that learning is basically recovery and recollection—that in the same way that bears and lions instinctively know everything they need to know to live and merely do it, each of us do, too. But, in our case, what we need to know gets lost in what we are told we should know."*
>
> Dennis Warren
> ***On Becoming a Leader***

Isn't that the truth . . . especially about food and our bodies. One of the first things we often do with clients is invite them to set aside their beliefs and allow some space for other possibilities.

Unlearning is often the basis for true understanding. Unlearning old food patterns is absolutely essential to discovering what foods, in what amounts, eaten at what times feel right for each of us.

The following activities are designed to help you recognize where you may be getting messages about what to eat and how chock-full of all these voices you are. You have little room to make sense of these messages, much less to hear the voice of your own intuition. Exploring is the first step of unlearning.

Hint: You may want to turn off the phone and television and find a quiet corner to complete this activity.

Imagine yourself in the TV section of a local appliance store surrounded with television screens full of talking heads—faces and voices blaring.

On one, a talk show host tells you to do what she has done for her weight; on another, a competing talk show host sells *her* approach to eating and health; on another, a model demonstrates weight loss exercises you ought to do. Don't miss the screen of your parents—their eyes rolling at even the thought of you wanting seconds of your favorite food. Of course, one screen has your co-workers discussing all the pounds they've lost on their latest regimes. Your spouse on the next screen reminds you what your body could be like—if you would just do what he or she does. Competing with these, a screen flashes a magazine listing of low-fat foods you should eat. The next screen babbles with an interview of a researcher about a new anti-food diet. And, finally, you fill in the rest of the screens with other messages you've received that we haven't suggested. Who else polices your food? What else pressures you to eat a certain way?

Now, surrounded with all the flashing screens and blaring voices, pick up the remote control, and, one by one, shut off each screen—*zap, zap, zap* . . .

With all the screens blank, take a moment just to feel the silence. This quiet space is where unlearning begins. This quiet is where *you* begin to discover and explore your own inner wisdom about food. This quiet is where you can begin to hear your *own* voice, rather than what the latest talking head tells you to do.

What foods make *me* feel satisfied? What amounts of different foods give *me* energy? When am *I* hungry?

We all have many opportunities to collect more and more voices and talking heads. It's so noisy and confusing we don't even notice one more . . . until we take time to be quiet.

This might sound simple. Yet, it is often scary to experience such silence and not have any direction or guidance about food. It's difficult to feel comfortable moving around in the uncharted territory of self-discovery. But, once you do, you will be able to decide from your inner knowing rather than from absorbing information.

Discovering What's Right For You

1   As you go through the next week, keep a list of each situation where you struggle with food (what kind, how much, what you thought you should or shouldn't have eaten).

Situation: _____

Describe Struggle: _____

_____

_____

Situation: _____

Describe Struggle: _____

_____

_____

Situation: _____

Describe Struggle: _____

_____

_____

Situation: _____

Describe Struggle: _____

_____

_____

(Use additional paper if you need more space)

2   For each of these situations, try to identify who or what was the source of messages that set up your struggle in that situation.

Message: _____
Source: _____

Message: _____
Source: _____

Message: _____
Source: _____

Message: _____
Source: _____

(Use additional paper if you need more space)

3   Keep a list of meals or eating situations that felt *good*
    (what kind of food, how much, when was it, how your
    body felt before, during, and after you ate).

Situation: _____

What made it feel good?: _____

_____

_____

Situation: _____

What made it feel good?: _____

_____

_____

Situation: _____

What made it feel good?: _____

_____

_____

Situation: _____

What made it feel good?: _____

_____

_____

4   Watch for other areas in which you might be looking for voices to tell you what your path is: what investments to make, what your beliefs are, what to do at work, how you should be feeling, which books and affirmations to read. Is there a similarity between how you respond to these voices and how you respond to voices about eating and food choices?

Other areas besides food that I listen to voices about what to do:

_____

_____

_____

_____

chapter

2 *Meeting and Greeting Your "Intuitive Eater"*

Now, after clearing all the voices and experiencing the empty silence, we often fill it again with all of the questions that continually haunt us.

"When it comes to food, I know what to do.
Why can't I just do it?"

"Why do my will power and motivation always seem
to disappear?"

"Should I be 'good' or just eat what I want?"

"Why is it when I eat what I really want, I can't stop?"

The answers to these questions lie within you, though you may have abandoned that knowledge or forgotten it. This is the basic premise of intuitive eating—that you, *and no one else*, knows what is best for you.

You wonder how you can serve as final authority when all around you are other people who appear to experience success in their relationships with food. *"Look,"* you may argue, *"their diet plans and exercise programs work. If only I could eat like those people eat, I'd no longer have problems with food."* *"After all,"* you ask yourself, *"how could I possibly know what is best for me given that*

I have failed again and again to come to terms with food, weight and body image?"

You're right, but only by half. Many people have discovered successful relationships with food. Their food plans and exercise regimens do work—for them. These people are at peace with what they eat. They have energy, and they feel good about how much they weigh. They have discovered what works—*for themselves.*

Not for *you*, but for themselves. That is the key, the critical difference. The food which leaves one person energized may leave you feeling lethargic. The meal which satisfies someone else may leave you empty. A diet plan which works for your neighbor or your co-worker may call for five starches a day, yet your body may require seven or eight, or only three. They've learned to understand their moods and feelings and how that affects what—and how much— they're wanting to eat. Furthermore, the amount of carbohydrate, protein or fat you need today may not be the same amount you'll need a week from today, a month from today, or next year. **Only you know what works for you:** what you need, in what amounts and when.

Prospective clients are always curious about what we will do for them and ask what program we will put them on. Our answer typically runs along the lines of, *"After we work with you to explore your history with food and your body, your beliefs about food and how bodies work, activity patterns, family needs, medical history, metabolic needs, schedules, food likes and dislikes, and your sense of where and how you fit in the world—who you are, where you're going, where you'd like to go, and your approach to living—we find a place to start. Then, we begin the process of tapping your intuitive eater."*

So, if you know already—if you are the expert—why do you continue to struggle with food? Where has your knowledge gone?

Silencing the Inner Intuitive Voice

Many people have lost contact with their intuitive knowledge regarding food. Everything in our culture tells us to ignore or to forget this vital inner knowledge.

Perhaps as a child you were urged, maybe even forced, to clean your plate when your body was not hungry. Perhaps you were made to eat foods your body did not like or need. Perhaps you were compelled to eat on a schedule which was not natural to you. Perhaps this happened often—regularly. In a variety of ways, many of us have learned that the instinctual way we felt about food was somehow flawed. Perhaps, too, the shape of your body did not please those you loved. Maybe people gave you messages which either further undermined your ability to trust yourself with your food choices, or made you feel guilty about eating in a way which you couldn't seem to control.

Events such as these encourage us not to trust ourselves. They teach us that others know what is best for us. Virtually all of our clients want us to tell them what is best for them. In response, we ask them lots of questions: what have they eaten, when, how much, how it felt, what else was going on with emotions, activity, schedules, are there similarities between their eating and other relationships and circumstances in life—even those as a child. Then, we review any nutrition principles that may apply to their needs—essentially helping them get used to hearing their body's signals and interpreting them so they can eventually answer the question themselves.

For some of us, the intuitive eater was healthy and vocal during childhood, only to have been silenced when we entered adolescence. Perhaps as your body changed, growing ever more mysterious and magical, the media images around you and the messages you received from family or peers were negative and hurtful. Perhaps you were told that your body was unacceptable and its appetites inappropriate. In all likelihood, by this time you had lost touch with your body and its needs. Perhaps you no longer tasted and enjoyed food, but had begun to fear it and to fight it.

If you are like many of our clients, you carried these patterns into adulthood and continued to experience failure in your relationship with food. By this time, the intuitive eater within lay asleep, thoroughly suppressed and nearly forgotten.

Now, let's start with the first powerful tools for waking up and re-energizing the helpful voice within.

Discovering What's Right For You

(Each of these activities asks you to notice signals on three levels: physical body signals, emotional feelings, and thoughts.)

1   Take a deep breath—so deep you can't take another breath. Hold your breath as long as you possibly can to a point where your body makes you breathe. Notice what signals your body starts to give you—any impulses you have—and the degrees to which you experience them. You have just experienced the "intuitive breather" within.

Body signals from your "intuitive breather"

_____

_____

_____

_____

_____

2   Do you have any recollections of similar experiences with eating where you took in more than was comfortable? What signals did the intuitive eater send you? Take a minute to remember any signals your body was giving you—sluggishness, dulled senses, stuffed feeling, nausea. Then notice your emotional responses and thoughts about what you did (for example—frustration, guilt, relief, surprise, elation, resignation, security).

Body signals
from eating too much

Emotional
responses
(example: frustration)

_____   _____
_____   _____
_____   _____
_____   _____
_____   _____
_____   _____
_____   _____

3   Do you remember any experiences when you ate too little? What happened to you? What were your body's signals that told you that you ate too little—headache, shaky, weak, irritable, recurring thoughts about food, nausea, light-headedness? Again, notice any thoughts or emotional responses.

Body signals   Emotional
from eating too little   responses
                                      (example: scared)

_____   _____
_____   _____
_____   _____
_____   _____
_____   _____
_____   _____
_____   _____
_____   _____

4   How does your body feel when you eat "just right?" Do
    you know what "just right" is? What physical sensations
    can you identify? What emotions do you feel? Calm, re-
    laxed, energized? Think of words to describe them.

Body signals   Emotional
from "just right" eating   responses
                                   (example: contented)

_____   _____
_____   _____
_____   _____
_____   _____
_____   _____
_____   _____
_____   _____

5   Practice listening to your intuitive eater. The next time you eat, notice any signals your body is giving you (physical, emotional, and mental) before, during and after you eat. List them.

Body signals

_____

_____
_____
_____
_____
_____

Don't worry if you don't pick up any signals at first. You'll get better at recognizing and feeling them as you do the exercises in this book.

Section Two:

Finding the Links

chapter

3

Listening to Body Signals

The chart below demonstrates the relationships of three brain chemicals (serotonin, endorphins, and dopamine) with emotions, moods, and food consumption. (Specific examples of foods that are high in starch, fat and protein are listed in Appendix I.)

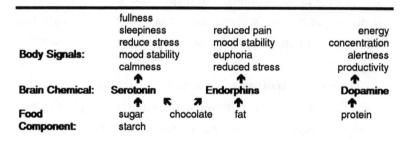

	fullness sleepiness reduce stress	reduced pain mood stability	energy concentration
Body Signals:	mood stability calmness ↑	euphoria reduced stress ↑	alertness productivity ↑
Brain Chemical:	**Serotonin** ↑ ↖ ↗	**Endorphins** ↑	**Dopamine** ↑
Food Component:	sugar chocolate starch	fat	protein

The Interaction Between Food and Brain Chemicals

Raised serotonin levels in the brain produce body signals of calm, relaxation, fullness, and perhaps sleepiness. When serotonin is low, we feel nervous, irritable, and stressed, and often have an appetite for carbohydrates or, more specifically, starches and sugars. This desire can be satisfied by food such as crackers, frozen yogurt, chocolate, chips, popcorn, candy bars, and rice cakes, to name a few of the more common options. Upon eating these foods, we usually experience a change in mood as a result of a rising concentration of serotonin and become relaxed, calm, and/or satisfied.

Don's case is a good example of how food, metabolism, and mental states are linked. The chief financial officer of a local film company, he frequently attends conferences and meetings. He wondered if he felt sleepy, foggy, and unable to concentrate because of what he ate at these events. Don came to us requesting help in creating a plan to feel better at these types of functions. He listed the typical fare: continental breakfast of sweet rolls or bagels and juice; breaks with cookies, muffins, or sodas; then, lunch buffets that included potatoes, rice, rolls, pasta, etc. After we reviewed with him the relationship between carbohydrates and serotonin levels, and how that affects sleepiness, we suggested he experiment by eating some protein in the morning, and then notice his body's reaction. He discovered that something as simple as having yogurt, a glass of milk, a piece of cheese or ham, or an egg seemed to prevent the foggy, sleepy feeling.

High concentrations of endorphins in the brain produce a sense of euphoria, enhance pleasure, and suppress pain, both emotionally and physically. When endorphins are low, people feel anxious; they are also more aware of pain. They have an appetite for fat and fatty foods, such as french fries, cheese, creamy sauces, margarine, butter, fried chicken, potato chips, and chocolate, to name some of the most popular examples. Upon eating some fat, they will notice a change in mood, feeling more pleasure. This feeling is related to a higher concentration of endorphins. Exercise, by releasing fat from within the body, raises endorphins and causes the same mood changes. Hence, moderate exercise can be an effective tool for controlling an appetite for fat.

Grace is experiencing a lot of pain from arthritis. As a result, she doesn't get out of the house much and often feels depressed and lonely. She complains of constantly battling with wanting fried foods and desserts all day—especially in the evenings. These foods are her only source of pleasure and she actually feels better physically after eating these. After she understood her current pattern in biochemical terms, she decided to try walking to see if burning her body's fat would supply the endorphins and pain relief she needed and reduce her desire for fatty foods. On days she is able to include some kind of movement, she has noticed that she has less intense cravings for fat.

Raised dopamine concentrations in the brain cause us to feel alert, focused, and energetic. When our dopamine levels are low, we may feel "foggy" and tend to have less ability to concentrate. Eating lean protein (lean roast beef or ham; turkey; grilled chicken; or fish), along with moderate amounts of carbohydrates and fats, raises dopamine concentrations most effectively; the result is increased alertness and concentration. Examples of meals that incorporate these elements are a lean roast beef or tuna sandwich with light mayonnaise, or a grilled chicken salad with a small amount of salad dressing and croutons or crackers. (For other meal ideas see Appendix II.)

Fred provides another example of how these principles work in real life. A manager for a popular band, he noticed that he felt clear and productive when he skipped breakfast and ate meats and vegetables for lunch. By the end of the day he felt agitated and hungry, and dove into boxes of crackers and bags of popcorn. Fred was feeling the effects of protein on dopamine levels early in the day (for energy and clarity), yet knew he was out of balance by late afternoon. Once he understood the food/brain chemistry link, he decided to experiment with adding carbohydrates throughout the day to reduce the feelings of agitation and stress. However, he still kept protein as the larger portion of his meals to retain the clarity and energy he needed.

One of many factors that constitute one's ideal meal is that it contains protein, carbohydrate, and fat, in proportions that will enable us to produce and maintain balance of brain chemicals. This, in turn, brings stability to moods and future food choices.

Discovering What's Right For You

See if you feel or recognize situations in your daily life similar to the ones just described that might have some relationship to amounts and timing of protein, carbohydrates, fats, or types of foods that you are eating. You may want to experiment as these people did to see if you feel any different with varying proportions of these foods.

Amount	Time	Protein	Sensations/Feelings

Amount	Time	Carbohydrate	Sensations/Feelings

Amount	Time	Fat	Sensations/Feelings

chapter

4

Recognizing Set-ups for Overeating — Emotional Cues

Frequently, people say they're eating for emotional reasons without fully understanding how or why this occurs. Many times we know what we should do. We know we'd feel better if we'd just eat a certain way. But, we wind up eating a few or a lot more cookies or rolls than we know we need for physical energy. In fact, sometimes we wind up feeling stuffed and full. Or, sometimes we don't eat—we can't. We're hungry but, somehow, food just won't go down. We *know* our body needs the food but we can't eat. We abandon our best intentions and most meticulous plans, best and most forceful expression of will power and most "abstinent" and perfectly followed food plans that have felt great and provided all kinds of energy, concentration, calmness—all in the right balance.

When that happens, look for emotional triggers, both chronic and short-term. Often, our responses are based on an accumulation of a lifetime of events, both struggles and pleasures. Most of the time, we are not even aware that certain past experiences are still influencing our current responses. At other times, it is easier to identify what may be influencing your response and why.

When things seem stressful, a cascade of hormones such as norepinephrine, epinephrine and adrenaline cause changes in dopamine and other brain chemicals producing a sense of anxiety and irritation. These are physically expressed by heart palpitations, tightness in your chest, flushing, panic attacks, spastic colon, irritable stomachs, diarrhea, constipation, teeth grinding, dry mouth, and headaches. If you are unable to or don't believe you can handle these feelings, you may choose to numb them either by over- or undereating. Remember the chart from Chapter 3 showing that the drive for sweets and sugars is a way to raise serotonin (a brain chemical) for more sedation and calmness; and a drive for fats is a way to raise endorphins (another brain chemical) for more pleasure. Raising the levels of these brain chemicals can help relieve the stress symptoms by balancing the high levels of dopamine and stress hormones.

On the other hand, undereating causes body fats to break down; which, in turn, creates high levels of endorphins, giving you some relief of stressful symptoms. Undereating also breaks down body proteins. This raises dopamine levels causing a "high"—a sense of power and protection from fear or a feeling of alertness and control.

As you can see, there *is* a direct link between what we're expressing emotionally and our physical bodies—our desire for food or certain foods and our lack of desire for food or certain ingredients in food.

The chemical changes caused by over- and undereating is one way we cope with feelings. Another is to continually focus on what we should be eating or not eating and what we weigh. This focus often keeps us locked into feeling shame, guilt, anger, disgust and hatred *at ourselves.* Which, in turn, "protects" us from dealing with the emotions, person, place or event that was the *real* source of our stress.

Another technique for not dealing with uncomfortable feelings is to focus on pampering yourself. Ironically, running from appointments with your therapist, nutritionist, massage therapist, skin specialist, personal trainer, etc., all in trying to take care of yourself, can also be a way to avoid feeling. This is not to say that pampering and basic self-care aren't important, just that *even* pampering can be used to avoid your feelings.

People who don't use food or other substances or addictions in the face of stress, have often learned other ways to handle uncomfortable feelings by talking about them, writing about them, and experiencing/exploring them in order to heal them. For many of these people, there is a confidence that they aren't going to be stuck in that feeling for the rest of their lives or die because of that feeling. They know it will pass and that they have tools to confront and take care of that feeling and comfort themselves. As a result of these beliefs, their brain chemistry changes are not as intense, which makes it easier to not use food to cope.

The ideas we've explored here may be very difficult to successfully explore and carry out on your own. For some ideas about finding support to help you address these, see Chapter 23.

Discovering What's Right For You

1   Identify situations—people, places, events—that trigger uncomfortable feelings and see if these have any effect on your eating patterns. Are there particular foods that you go for?

Trigger Situations for uncomfortable feelings (Example: people, locations, events)	Effect on eating	Certain foods
_____	_____	_____
_____	_____	_____
_____	_____	_____
_____	_____	_____
_____	_____	_____
_____	_____	_____
_____	_____	_____
_____	_____	_____

2   Identify if you have any eating pattern or food choices linked with positive emotions and events—excitement, celebration, anticipation.

Situations that you enjoy	Effect on eating	Certain foods
_____	_____	_____
_____	_____	_____
_____	_____	_____
_____	_____	_____
_____	_____	_____
_____	_____	_____
_____	_____	_____

3   List any physical sensations you notice, which lets you
    know you are feeling, i.e. headaches, butterflies in your
    stomach, knots or pain in your stomach. Sometimes we
    don't even notice we're feeling the emotions, but we can
    pick up a physical sensation that may represent an emo-
    tional feeling.

Physical sensations noticed during situations from 1 and 2 above

_____

_____

_____

_____

_____

_____

4   Notice how you feel after you've used food to cope with
    feelings by either under or over eating. Do you feel numb
    or enlivened, calmed or stuffed, raw, disgusted with your-
    self? What else?

Overeating causes: feelings and sensations

_____

_____

_____

Undereating causes: feelings and sensations

_____

_____

_____

5   If you ate after a particular feeling or event, can you iden-
    tify anything besides the food that you really wanted in-
    stead? What needs, if any, weren't being met? (Did you
    want attention, a hug, to be left alone, etc.?) Don't be sur-
    prised if, in response to this question, you draw a blank.
    Rarely do we give ourselves permission to even think
    about what it is we really want. If this is the case, you may
    want to start listing any needs that you can identify.

    What did I really want or need, other than food,
     during the situations recorded in questions 1 and 2?

    _____

    _____

    _____

5 *Recognizing Set-ups for Overeating — Physiological Cues*

Those of us who occasionally experience cravings and those who struggle with chronic out-of-control eating experience physical set-ups that intensify appetites. Often, physical cravings are the body's way of trying to get its needs met. This chapter lists some of the physical conditions affecting appetite.

⇒ A well-fueled average-size body stores about 100–300 grams of carbohydrate to supply the body's energy needs. In addition, these stores keep hunger at bay for about 4–5 hours before depleting to a point where hunger starts becoming intense. When people don't eat enough carbohydrate, their bodies will set up a physically intense drive to crave it. Then when they eat carbohydrate, their hunger will diminish.

⇒ When carbohydrate stores are depleted, the body begins to break down muscle protein for fuel. As a result of muscle breakdown, stress hormones are released into the blood and brain. These hormones turn on appetite for carbohydrate. These stress hormones are also released when you feel emotional stress and similarly cause an increase in appetite for carbohydrate.

⇒ Protein plays an important part in controlling appetite. Adequate amounts of protein eaten with carbohydrate help moderate the rate at which carbohydrate is absorbed into the blood stream. As a result, hunger is controlled. Without adequate protein, the body's appetite for carbohydrate is much more intense and frequent because it is absorbed from the stomach faster, leaving the stomach empty, which triggers signals of hunger.

⇒ Lack of exercise results in low levels of endorphins (pleasure hormones) which, in turn, may set up cravings for fat which helps raise endorphins. (See Chapter 3 chart.)

⇒ Also, intensity of exercise can set up cravings and cause overeating—usually on carbohydrate. The more intense the exercise, the greater the likelihood that you will deplete your carbohydrate stores. And, as said above, low carbohydrate stores cause hunger for starches and sugars. The more moderate the exercise, the less intense the appetite for carbohydrate.

⇒ Appetite is also affected by our senses. A variety of tastes, textures, smells, colors, temperatures, and density of foods satisfy pleasure centers in the brain. If we feed ourselves based on our body's signals, we will satisfy these pleasure centers and turn off appetite. If we chronically deprive our pleasure centers we will feel a hunger for foods which our experience has taught us will satisfy these centers.

Suggestions to explore your physiological cues to overeat are listed at the end of the next chapter. We encourage you to read Chapter 6 before attempting these activities.

6

Craving Sweets and Starches

If you don't eat enough carbohydrate you're going to crave it. This is not about having enough willpower. It is about going with your gut, your intuitive eater.

Before you panic, we are *not* encouraging you to dive into sacks and sacks of doughnuts. In fact, this kind of binge is often a result of ignoring your intuitive eater. Instead, we are going to help you understand where such an urge comes from, the signals that your intuitive eater sends you, and how to prevent your cravings.

Each body requires a certain level of carbohydrate to function: for muscle activity, brain activity, sleep-wake cycles, mood stability, appetite control—all day, all night. The amount and timing of carbohydrate needed for each individual will vary according to body size, amount of muscle tissue, heredity, climate, season of the year, activity, intensity of activity, etc. Because of all these variables, no one but your intuitive eater can tell you exactly what your carbohydrate needs are.

Night Binges: The Intuitive Eater Screams

Do you ever wonder why you feel out of control with your carbohydrate eating at night after you've been so diligent all through the day—controlling every morsel that passes your lips? You've had half of a grapefruit and a slice of diet toast, a can of water-pack tuna for lunch with a few carrots. Then the five o'clock munchies hit, evolving into an evening-long binge on chips, ice cream, cookies, candy, and brownies.

You have just experienced your intuitive eater screaming, *"I need carbs!"* Amazingly, it had whispered to you sometime earlier in the day, continuing with greater intensity throughout the day. But, you were determined to override it until it got so loud that you couldn't bear it. Your willpower had to give in. You were out of control—again.

If you've ever experienced this, you can be confident your intuitive eater is there, alive, well and talking to you . . . and that you are not listening.

How does it speak to you? What sensations does it whisper or shout to you? Ripples in your stomach, sensations in your mouth, gurgles in your stomach, aches, waves of aches or weakness, fuzzy or scattered thinking? Different people experience it in different ways.

If you listen and respond by eating meals and snacks that include enough carbohydrate when it starts to talk, it won't have to shout and you won't have to binge. In this case, the intuitive eater starts whispering when biochemically, your muscles run out of carbohydrate energy, your blood sugar is low and your brain serotonin levels fall. What it's asking you to do is refuel. As these get emptier and emptier, the body releases hormones and other brain chemicals that make the intuitive eater more insistent and louder.

Sugar Cravings

Often you won't interpret the urge to eat sugar as *"I need car-bohydrate."* Instead, you'll hear *"I need sweets."* The reasons:

⇒ A can of cola or a 2-oz. candy bar has as much carbohydrate as a baked potato or a cup of rice. Sugar is a very concen-trated source of carbohydrate. So, your *panicked* intuitive eater knows it can get more of what it needs in fewer bites with sugar.

⇒ Sugar is more quickly digested and absorbed than other car-bohydrates. When your intuitive eater is desperate for fuel, your taste buds crave the sweet flavors and textures of sugars. This way, it gets the carbohydrates it needs much faster than it would from other carbohydrate-rich foods. That's why you choose ice cream, candy, soft drinks, and cookies. You can prevent this act of desperation from happening by listen-ing to your intuitive eater earlier.

⇒ Sugar is easy to eat and more accessible. How many vending machines have rice, potatoes, bread, or corn on the cob? Even if they did, where would you cook it or sit down to eat it? These foods are just not as portable and convenient as sugar and sweets.

Don't Forget Protein

The minute clients start describing their struggle with not be-ing able to stop eating chips, crackers, bread, rice, cereal, ice cream, cookies, and carbohydrate-rich foods, we start searching for protein in their meals and snacks. Often, it will show up in a half-cup of milk on their cereal, one wafer-thin slice of turkey on their sandwich, or a sprinkle of cheese on their salad or spaghetti.

This is a whopping 10 grams of protein from protein-rich foods. Most bodies need at least 40, if not 60–100 grams each day. (See the activities section at the end of this chapter to help you de-termine how much protein you need each day.)

Why do we look for protein when people struggle with overeating? Consider that:

⇒ adequate amounts of protein spread throughout the day can minimize the intensity of food cravings. A building block of protein is tryptophan, which along with carbohydrate, creates the brain chemical serotonin. Remember, serotonin in the right amounts flips the craving switch off.

⇒ including protein in each meal will help people feel full longer because it takes longer to be absorbed from the stomach and it slows down the absorption of carbohydrate. Many people who struggle with hypoglycemia and sugar cravings often find this helpful. Another advantage of eating protein is that dopamine, the brain chemical raised by protein, helps people feel more alert, productive, and better able to concentrate.

Good protein-rich food sources are lean meats, poultry, fish, shellfish, eggs, egg substitutes, milk (most rice and soy milks are not good sources), yogurt (not frozen yogurt), cheese (not cream cheese), beans, tofu, tempeh, and nutritional yeast.

While many people believe that they can get their protein needs met by eating carbohydrate-rich foods—bread, cereal, crackers, rice, potatoes, pasta, pretzels and popcorn at 2–3 grams in each serving—they would have to eat about 30 servings of these carbohydrate-rich foods (about 3000 calories) to meet their protein needs.

Most people would be eating more carbohydrate than they need using this approach. If you feel omitting protein-rich foods and bingeing on carbohydrates is what you're doing, it may be that your body is trying to get the protein it needs from carbohydrate-rich foods.

Cravings: One More Reason

If you notice that you feel more alert, more in control, and much less hungry on days with no carbohydrates than on days you ate carbohydrates throughout the day, you are not weird. Your intuitive eater is letting you know what is a good match for your system. You simply have a system that runs differently than what most nutrition columns, magazine articles, and health professionals are writing about. Don't worry, you are not alone. It is estimated that a quarter of the American population have systems that run in this way. No wonder these folks are frustrated. They are trying to follow recommendations made for the other 75% of the population!

We see many people who, in trying to be good, force themselves to override their intuitive eater and follow recommendations to eat lots of carbohydrate, only to feel more and more out of control. We frequently see this in people who: have a family history of diabetes, are relatively inactive, feel *more* hungry when they eat breakfast than when they don't, crave carbohydrates, have high blood fats, and often have a large proportion of fat cells to lean cells in their body. These are indicators of insulin resistance—when your body's cells don't allow insulin to open cells up to allow carbohydrate to flow in.

This sets up carbohydrate cravings because your muscle cells and brain are not receiving the carbohydrates and don't know that you've eaten them. The liver then takes this extra carbohydrate that isn't being absorbed and converts it to fat for storage. Hence the high blood fats and increasing fat weight despite your best efforts to eat "right" by eating lots of carbohydrate and no fat.

So, what can you do? One of the easiest ways to work with this type of system, alter its ability to use carbohydrates, and minimize carbohydrate cravings is to have some form of exercise, daily. Exercise makes the cells in your body more receptive to the insulin.

But, you will still need to make some changes in the way you eat. This is where your intuitive eater will be helpful. Eating much more protein and much less carbohydrate than normally recommended is usually helpful in controlling hunger and cravings and usually stops weight gain. Listening to your intuitive eater is essential to determine how much protein and carbohydrates to eat and when to eat them during the day. The exercises that follow will help you determine this.

Discovering What's Right For You

These activities are not going to give you an answer right away, or in one or two tries. Many of you who have ignored your intuitive eater for a very long time should plan to repeat this activity over and over to have a more finely tuned ear for your intuitive eater.

1   Try avoiding carbohydrate-rich foods for the first eight hours of one day. Keep a list of any sensations your body experiences. After the eight hours are over, eat carbohydrate-rich foods and note your sensations.

Sensations during 8 hrs. of no carbohydrates

_____

_____

_____

Sensations after eating carbohydrates after your 8-hour test

_____

_____

_____

2   Try having one or two servings of carbohydrate-rich foods
    at breakfast and at lunch for two or three days and note the
    signals and intensity of the signals and the intensity of any
    craving at night, if any.

Sensations after 1-2 servings of carbohydrate at breakfast

Day 1	Day 2	Day 3
_____	_____	_____
_____	_____	_____
_____	_____	_____

Sensations after 1-2 servings of carbohydrate at lunch

Day 1	Day 2	Day 3
_____	_____	_____
_____	_____	_____
_____	_____	_____

3   Then, for another 2–3 days double the amount of
    carbohydrate-rich foods eaten at each meal and note the
    signals your body and intuitive eater give you.

Sensations after 2-4 servings of carbohydrate at breakfast

Day 1	Day 2	Day 3
_____	_____	_____
_____	_____	_____
_____	_____	_____

Sensations after 2-4 servings of carbohydrate at lunch

Day 1	Day 2	Day 3
_____	_____	_____
_____	_____	_____
_____	_____	_____

4   What's the right amount of protein for you and how do you fit it into your meals? First, you may want to record what you're eating for a day or two and note which foods are rich in protein.

Day 1	Day 2	✓ protein-rich foods (use appendix 1)
_____	_____	_____
_____	_____	_____
_____	_____	_____
_____	_____	_____
_____	_____	_____
_____	_____	_____
_____	_____	_____
_____	_____	_____
_____	_____	_____
_____	_____	_____
_____	_____	_____
_____	_____	_____
_____	_____	_____
_____	_____	_____
_____	_____	_____
_____	_____	_____
_____	_____	_____
_____	_____	_____
_____	_____	_____
_____	_____	_____
_____	_____	_____
_____	_____	_____
_____	_____	_____
_____	_____	_____

5   Experiment with eating a meal or two with no protein-rich foods. For example, eat a vegetable salad and rolls, pasta with meatless marinara sauce, or a vegetable plate. Notice when you get hungry again after the meal. Now, compare that to another day when you eat a restaurant-size portion of protein-rich foods (about 4–6 ounces of cooked meat or 1–2 cups of beans, for example). Which meal makes you feel full longer? [Note: Carbohydrate is sometimes a variable in this too. If you aren't getting a clear test on this, you may want to see a nutritionist for an evaluation of your approximate protein and carbohydrate needs and how to be able to use labels to help determine this.]

No protein meal

Foods	How long until you felt hungry	Sensations of hunger after meal

Restaurant-size portion of protein meal

Foods	How long until you felt hungry	Sensations of hunger after meal

6 Using the same experiment, notice if you're sleepy or more alert, and any effect on your ability to concentrate with these different meals.

Non-protein meal
from above:

(circle one)

sleepy   alert

Comments about concentration

_____

_____

_____

Protein-rich meal
from above:

(circle one)

sleepy   alert

Comments about concentration

_____

_____

_____

7 Repeat the same experiment and notice if protein-rich meals affect cravings later in the day. Compare this to no-protein or low-protein meals.

No/low-protein meal

Effect on cravings

_____

_____

_____

Protein-rich meal

Effect on cravings

_____

_____

_____

8 Repeat these experiments as many times as you need to begin to feel confident that, on a daily basis, your intuitive eater talks to you and sends different signals depending on how much carbohydrate and protein you eat and when you eat it.

You may want to get a notebook to keep notes about the effects of protein-rich and non-protein meals over the next several days or weeks. Jot some notes here if you'd like.

9 Experiment with your first meal of the day. Eat only protein and vegetables. To make sure this is a good test, start
   with at least six units of protein. (See appendix.) Some examples are: two chicken breasts, six eggs or egg substitutes
   (don't worry about the cholesterol here, this is just for the
   experiment), a 6-oz. lean steak, 1–1½ cups of cottage
   cheese or any combination of protein-rich foods as listed
   in the appendix. Add vegetables if you'd like. Notice how
   long this meal keeps you full and track any other signals
   your intuitive eater is giving you.

   The next day, make your first meal mostly carbohydrate-rich foods—enough for you to be pleasantly full,
   but not stuffed—maybe as much as 4–6 servings. (See Appendix 1.) You may include fruits and fruit juices in addition to the carbohydrate-rich sugars and starches. Again,
   notice how long this meal keeps you full.

   What are the differences in how your body feels after the
   protein meal and after the carbohydrate meal?

Protein-rich first meal of the day   _____
Time you ate: _____
Time you noticed hunger: _____

Carbohydrate-rich first meal of the day _____
Time you ate: _____
Time you noticed hunger: _____

10 We'd like to challenge you to test the effect of *moderate* daily exercise (see Chapter 12) on your carbohydrate cravings. Keep notes on how you feel. These changes will be more subtle and will happen over a longer period of time—two to three weeks.

Hold on to your notes because this only begins to unlock what your intuitive eater does. You'll gather more information from other chapters about how other things affect it.

Kind of exercise	Minutes	Effect on hunger / cravings
_____	_____	_____
_____	_____	_____
_____	_____	_____
_____	_____	_____

7

Cravings and PMS

There is a physical, biochemical reason why many women increase their intake of sugar, fat, and chocolate just prior to, or early in, their menstrual periods.

Below, we discuss highlights of the underlying physiology of PMS and how it affects food cravings and list some suggestions for minimizing food cravings and the physical discomforts often associated with PMS.

You may recall from Chapter 3 that high carbohydrate consumption (starches and sugars) along with small amounts of protein help to increase serotonin levels in the brain, which results in calm and satiated feelings. Exercise and eating fats and chocolate help raise endorphin levels in the brain, which increase feelings of pleasure and reduce pain.

Female hormones can also influence serotonin and endorphin levels and thereby, the appetite for certain food components. As hormones fluctuate during the monthly cycle, the levels of serotonin and endorphins also fluctuate. The chart below demonstrates this relationship.

After Period	Ovulation	Prior to Period	
↑ serotonin	↑ endorphins	↓ estrogen	↑ progesterone
↑ estrogen		↓ serotonin	↑ pain & tenderness
		↓ endorphins	↑ irritability

Estrogen levels are higher in the first two weeks of the monthly cycle and have a direct influence on increasing serotonin levels. Progesterone is highest in the last two weeks of the cycle and tends to break down serotonin. Endorphin levels increase mid-cycle. Within two to three days after ovulation, endorphin levels begin to drop due to rising levels of progesterone. The drop in estrogen and rise in progesterone cause a greater appetite for fat and sugar due to their effects on serotonin and endorphins. For reasons still unknown, some women have larger fluctuations in these hormones (estrogen and progesterone) and therefore in neurotransmitters (serotonins and endorphins) than other women. Wide fluctuations can exacerbate difficulties with food during PMS (overeating, restricting consumption, unhealthy food choices, etc.).

Some tips to minimize the impact of these fluctuations are offered below.

For raising serotonin:

♦ Increase consumption of complex carbohydrate/starchy foods (breads, flours, pastas, dried peas, and beans). Amounts and timing of increases vary according to individual needs.

♦ Consume little or no sugar. If you do have sugar, make sure it is combined with other foods (i.e. in a meal with starches, high fiber foods and/or protein rich foods) so that blood sugar swings are diminished.

◆ Eat small meals or snacks at frequent intervals to provide a constant source of carbohydrates (and perhaps some protein) to stabilize levels of neurotransmitters.

◆ Vitamin B6 must be present for the body to produce serotonin. Consuming foods rich in B6 (such as dried beans and peas, whole grains, and meats) and other B vitamins often enhances the production of serotonin. For others, a B6 supplement is required to reduce food cravings and prevent physical discomfort. You may need to talk to your nutritionist or physician if you plan to take a B6 supplement to determine the correct dosage.

For raising endorphins:

◆ Moderate fat consumption. For some, this may mean adding some extra fat to a usual pattern of low fat consumption during the weeks prior to the period.

◆ Include moderate aerobic exercise to break down body fats which will reduce the craving for fats. *Don't* omit protein as this is necessary for providing some of the building blocks for serotonin and endorphins.

These are just **some** of the major nutritional elements to consider when addressing PMS symptoms. Addressing just one element is often ineffective. For example, you could have plenty of carbohydrates but not the necessary B6 or protein, resulting in continuing symptoms. Therefore, it may be useful to document your food intake and exercise patterns and consult with a qualified nutritionist to find what adjustments, if any, may work best for you.

chapter

8

Controlling Appetite — Other Variables

People often say, *"My intuitive eater wants me to binge on hamburgers or milkshakes or both!"* But, as you practice working with your intuitive eater, you will be able to distinguish the signal of a true physical need for hamburgers from an emotional response to some experience, or your rebel trying to get your attention to protect you from something it fears.

Many factors influence our desire for food. Two of the most well understood pathways for preventing cravings we discussed in Chapters 3 and 4. There are probably thousands of other pathways in the body which also affect or are affected by food. We don't even need to know all the details of how these pathways work to be able to use them effectively because our intuitive eater communicates with these pathways and signals to us what we need to know.

Below we've listed some of the pathways of which we are currently aware. We present them here to illustrate the amazing complexity and resources that the human body has at its disposal to "feel," respond and direct the body, unconsciously, to meet its needs.

CCK (cholecystokinin). CCK is a powerful appetite regulator released in the small intestine by the presence of fat and protein. It is believed that it slows down stomach emptying and sends signals to the brain that cause that "can't-eat-another-bite" sensation. So, when a meal or snack includes protein and fat, your body releases CCK and helps you feel full faster. Some people may have more CCK than others or at certain emotional periods in their life they may secrete more in response to the emotion. These people may feel hungry, but fill up very quickly. On the other hand, some people may not secrete much or be less sensitive to the CCK they secrete, thereby needing more food to feel "full."

Galanin. The body has a built-in appetite control system for fat which is, in part, influenced by galanin. The more galanin produced the greater the appetite for fat. The hormone estrogen can activate galanin. Women, particularly those with a high percentage of their weight in fat, produce more estrogen than women with a lower percentage body fat. Therefore, women who have higher body fat generally eat more fat than women with less body fat.

Neuropeptide Y. Our hunger for carbohydrate can be stimulated by neuropeptide Y. It is switched on after any long period of not eating or by the release of stress hormones. Skipping meals, overriding hunger, vigorous activity, having someone yell at you, having a fender bender in your car, having more bills due than money to pay them—all of these stimulate release of neuropeptide Y and thus, an appetite for carbohydrates.

Seasons. Some people's appetites are more sensitive than others to effects of the amount and length of time exposed to daylight. Natural daylight enables the body to produce melatonin, a hormone, which helps induce sleep. With shorter days and less daylight, much of the melatonin needed is produced from serotonin (rather than light). This reduces the levels of serotonin in the brain which turns on hunger for carbohydrates. (See Chapter 3.) Some people seem to over-produce melatonin in winter months. This condition is called Seasonal Affective Disorder (SAD). These people tend to want to just eat-and-sleep. The more they sleep, the more melatonin and serotonin they use *and* the more they want to eat, especially sugar and starchy foods, to replace the depleted serotonin.

Cortisol. This hormone is produced by the body during stress and has a particular propensity to turn on the taste for carbohydrate by revving up the production of Neuropeptide Y.

Glucagon. Glucagon is the opposing hormone to insulin. That is, it does the opposite of insulin. Insulin helps cells store carbohydrate. When insulin and carbohydrate levels are low, glucagon is released into the blood stream to pull the stored carbohydrates back into the blood stream. This helps to decrease appetite. In addition, high protein meals help stimulate glucagon release, as does exercise. This is the reason why immediately after exercise, many people have little appetite.

Estrogen. The female hormone, estrogen, stimulates increased production of galanin and, as a result, increases desire for fat. The irony here is that the more body fat a woman has, the more estrogen she secretes.

Social situations. Research suggests that we are 28% more hungry when we eat with one companion than when we eat alone and that we have 76% greater appetite when eating with six or more people. On the other hand, many of our clients notice they eat much less when they are with others and feel freer and less ashamed to eat large volumes when alone.

Gender. Other research shows women tend to overeat when lonely and depressed, while men more often overeat in social situations, or when feeling happy.

Genes. Certain people genetically have fat cells that secrete greater amounts of hormones that act in the brain to increase or decrease appetite. Others have brain cells that are genetically more receptive or less receptive to these hormones. Addressing the variables we've discussed in this book often minimizes the intensity of the impact of these genetic conditions. In much the same way that people who are genetically predisposed to type II adult onset diabetes or hypercholesterolemia can prevent, delay the onset of, or minimize its consequences by their living and eating patterns, so, too, can people minimize genetic influences on appetite and weight by applying the information in this book and paying attention to and responding to body signals.

Genes and Taste. Taste plays a big role in what people eat. Researchers suggest that the whole world can be split into three categories—non-tasters, tasters, and super-tasters—depending on the intensity and the way they perceive bitterness, sweetness and other taste sensations. Foods like broccoli, brussel sprouts, and mustard greens, which are naturally bitter, can seem unpleasantly so to some because of the taste genes people inherit. Women are more likely than men to be super-tasters, and Asians and blacks are more apt than whites to have this trait. In general, studies show: super-tasters are apparently more sensitive to tastes because they have more taste buds on their tongues; super-tasters are more likely to find bitter foods to be nastily bitter and sweet things to be cloyingly sweet (dairy fat tastes creamier, chili peppers are hotter and carbonated drinks may be unpleasantly bubbly); non-tasters are likely to say saccharin tastes fine, while super-tasters find an unpleasant aftertaste; female super-tasters are less likely to be obese and appear to have better cholesterol levels—furthermore, they seem to enjoy cooking more.

Other research has shown that people can eat a plate full of chips, for example, feel full, and stop. But when they see a different food, maybe nuts or grapes, neurons in the brain start firing impulses that attract them to this new taste and encourages them to start eating again despite their hunger level.

Liver metabolism. When the liver experiences being fed with glucose or fat and that is paired with eating a particular food, people develop a liking for that food. One study showed that men developed a liking for spinach when researchers infused their livers with glucose while being fed spinach.

Emotional pairing. Often you will hear someone say nothing tastes as good as their mother's apple pie. They prefer *their* mother's pie to anyone else's. It is theorized that the hormonal changes associated with good feelings and brain impressions made at the time they were experiencing the tastes and textures of their mother's pie literally make a lasting impression that no other apple pie can quite duplicate.

Sometimes, people will search for that impression and feeling by consuming similar foods, yet never be quite satisfied. Likewise, food eaten when a person is nauseated or during an unpleasant physical or emotional experience can result in a lasting aversion to that food. For that reason, it is suggested that food should never be forced upon people, especially children, and that meal-time be a time for pleasure and true nurturance.

As you can see, there are many ways our bodies regulate appetite. Your intuitive eater is an invaluable tool for using all of these systems to feel full and fulfilled.

Discovering What's Right For You

1   Keep a food and activity journal. Review the journal noting where some of the appetite regulators listed below may be playing a role in your food choices. Examples: For glucagon, if you have a particularly vigorous workout, notice your appetite 5–10 minutes after you complete your exercise. For Neuropeptide Y, notice your appetite one-to-four hours after a vigorous workout (assuming you have no food during this time). What do you want? What are you drawn to?

CCK (cholecystokinin):

Galanin:

Neuropeptide Y:

Seasons:

Cortisol:

Glucagon:

Estrogen:

Social Situations:

Gender:

Genes:

Genes and Taste:

Liver Metabolism:

Emotional Pairing:

Serotonin:

Endorphins:

Dopamine:

Exercise:

9 *Relating Body Composition to Appetite and Hunger*

Having your body composition measured is not required for eating intuitively. However, recognizing how it affects intuitive eating is important.

Basically, body weight is divided into two major components: lean tissue weight and fat tissue weight. Lean weight includes muscle, carbohydrate stores in muscle and the liver, water that is stored in the body, blood, bone, and all the components of the body that are not fat. Fat weight is essentially all fat: in muscle, around organs, and under the skin.

A pound of fat contains 3,500 calories, but a pound of lean tissue contains approximately 500 calories. If the scale indicates an increase or decrease of a pound, there is no way to tell whether the change is fat or lean. However, if a change of 2 or 3 lbs. occurs in a couple of days, we can demonstrate by doing the math that one would have to burn 7–10,000 extra calories to lose fat, or eat 7–10,000 extra calories to gain fat. A change of 2 or 3 lbs. of lean tissue (muscle, carbohydrates, water, etc.), on the other hand, involves only 1,000–1,500 calories, which is a much more likely amount to change in a couple of days. For reasons described below, losing lean tissue is detrimental and can cause lack of energy, increased hunger and cravings.

The examples below compare two people with different amounts of lean tissue and the same amount of activity.

Individual 1
200 lbs. total body weight

   50 lbs. fat
  150 lbs. lean (muscle and bone)

1000 calorie carbohydrate storage capacity

Individual 2
200 lbs. total body weight

  100 lbs. fat
  100 lbs. lean (muscle and bone)

750 calorie carbohydrate storage capacity

Individual 1 has more lean tissue, therefore:

- has a greater capacity to burn fat because metabolism occurs in lean tissue.
- has a greater capacity to eat fat without gaining fat because of the higher metabolism.
- can store more carbohydrates (in muscle and liver.)
- can potentially eat bigger portions of carbohydrates in one sitting and not gain fat because of more muscle to store it in.
- experiences hunger less frequently because more muscle can store more carbohydrate.
- can do more activity without running out of energy because carbohydrates supply energy and this body can store more because of the greater amount of lean.

Individual 2 has less lean tissue, therefore:

♦ can store less carbohydrate, so can't eat as much carbohydrate in one sitting without gaining fat.

♦ experiences hunger more frequently because this person
can't store as much carbohydrate.

♦ will become fatigued sooner with the same amount of activity as the first individual because this one cannot store as
much carbohydrate.

♦ has less capacity to burn fat because less lean tissue means
lower metabolic rate.

♦ can't eat as much fat as Individual 1 without gaining fat because of a lower metabolic rate.

These points explain why diet programs generally fail. If the
two people above followed the same diet plan, one could gain fat
while another could lose fat. One could be hungrier much more often than the other. Rarely do programs use a person's body composition to determine and individualize food choices, quantities of
food, or timing of meals, nor do they consider body composition's
effects on appetite, energy, and mood.

Often, as a result, your intuitive eater starts screaming, making
it very difficult to continue following the plan. It sets up shame and
the belief, *"I don't have enough willpower,"* when in reality, your
intuitive eater is telling you about what it needs to supply your body
with a more accurate match to feel full and fulfilled.

So, if you have ever felt awful on a diet plan (hungry, craving,
tired), you now know your intuitive eater is active and trying to help.

Discovering What's Right For You

1   If there is a gym or hospital wellness center close by it might be interesting to have your body composition measured. If body fat is above 30% total body weight then you may particularly benefit from small infrequent meals.

Date   _____

body composition   _____

weight (pounds)   _____

pounds of fat tissue
(weight x %)   _____

pounds of lean tissue
(total weight—pounds of fat)   _____

2   If you experience frequent and/or intense hunger in spite of three large meals, try to spread out the same amount of food into three smaller meals and two to three snacks each day.

Experiment with smaller meals more often

Day 1	Day 2	Day 3

Record the times you were hungry

Day 1	Day 2	Day 3

chapter

10

Evaluating Success: The 1-2 Pound Trap

Have you fallen into the 1–2 pound per week trap? If you're not losing this much weight each week, do you feel like a failure? The following facts may help you re-evaluate what you use as a measure of success.

⇒ One pound of muscle or lean tissue has about 500 calories of carbohydrate and/or protein. One pound of fat has 3500 calories of fat.

⇒ It's easy to gain and/or lose the 500 calories of carbohydrate and protein because over half the calories you burn in one day are carbohydrate calories. If you burn 2000 calories per day and eat no carbohydrate, then you would lose almost two pounds (of lean tissue). Remember, though, from Chapter 9, there is no advantage to losing muscle.

⇒ For those of you who are fat gram counters, the 3500 calories contained in one pound of fat equals about 400 grams of fat.

⇒ The person eating a diet moderately low in fat and exercising regularly may lose anywhere from 10–40 grams of fat per day depending on the amount of lean tissue available to burn fat, how active they are, eating patterns, and many other variables.

⇒ In the best case scenario—with the greatest consistency of eating and exercise possible—a person could possibly lose a pound of fat in 10–40 days; that's very different from the expectation of losing 1–2 pounds per week.

⇒ The person who loses 1–2 pounds/week is most likely burning lean tissue, the tissue used to burn fat.

⇒ Daily weighing—even weekly weighing—is rarely a measure of fat burned and, as a result, is unproductive and de-motivating (given the fact that it takes 10–40 days to lose one pound of fat).

We suggest using some markers other than the scale to evaluate success such as:

♦ Do your meals pleasantly satisfy you throughout the day?

♦ Are you pleasantly hungry right before the next meal and pleasantly satisfied at the end of a meal or snack?

♦ Do you have plenty of energy throughout the day?

♦ Are you making new discoveries about food and exercise?

♦ Is your relationship with food changing? Are you finding new ways of getting satisfied without going to extremes?

♦ Are you developing more comfortable rhythms of eating and exercise?

♦ Are you beginning to develop new food choices or combinations that feel right?

♦ Are you reacting differently in your food, exercise and eating patterns when stress increases or when you have more time to yourself?

If you're interested in creating some new markers that work uniquely for you, make an appointment with a nutritionist who specializes in intuitive eating concepts.

Discovering What's Right For You

Experiment with some markers other than the scale to evaluate success.

1 For one day, notice if your meals pleasantly satisfy you throughout the day. What body signals did your intuitive eater send to let you know you were satisfied? Are you pleasantly hungry right before the next meal? What body signals did your intuitive eater send to let you know you were not satisfied?

Meal: _____

Signals of satisfaction: _____

_____

Signals of dissatisfaction: _____

_____

Meal: _____

Signals of satisfaction: _____

_____

Signals of dissatisfaction: _____

_____

Meal: _____

Signals of satisfaction: _____

_____

Signals of dissatisfaction: _____

_____

2   Track your energy level each day for a week. Notice how it is related to what, when, and how much you eat.

Day 1

Food   Energy Level

_____   _____

_____   _____

_____   _____

_____   _____

_____   _____

_____   _____

_____   _____

_____   _____

_____   _____

Day 2

Food   Energy Level

_____   _____

_____   _____

_____   _____

_____   _____

_____   _____

_____   _____

_____   _____

_____   _____

_____   _____

Day 3

Food	Energy Level
_____	_____
_____	_____
_____	_____
_____	_____
_____	_____
_____	_____
_____	_____
_____	_____
_____	_____
_____	_____

Day 4

Food	Energy Level
_____	_____
_____	_____
_____	_____
_____	_____
_____	_____
_____	_____
_____	_____
_____	_____
_____	_____

Day 5

Food	Energy Level
_____	_____
_____	_____
_____	_____
_____	_____
_____	_____
_____	_____
_____	_____
_____	_____
_____	_____
_____	_____
_____	_____
_____	_____
_____	_____

Day 6

Food	Energy Level
_____	_____
_____	_____
_____	_____
_____	_____
_____	_____
_____	_____
_____	_____
_____	_____
_____	_____
_____	_____
_____	_____
_____	_____

Day 7

Food	Energy Level
_____	_____
_____	_____
_____	_____
_____	_____
_____	_____
_____	_____
_____	_____
_____	_____
_____	_____
_____	_____
_____	_____
_____	_____

Day 8

Food	Energy Level
_____	_____
_____	_____
_____	_____
_____	_____
_____	_____
_____	_____
_____	_____
_____	_____
_____	_____
_____	_____
_____	_____

3   Are you making new discoveries about food and exercise?
    For example, are you bingeing less, enjoying meals more,
    panicking less when making decisions about eating and/or
    exercise, etc.?

    Other markers of progress and discoveries:

    _____
    _____
    _____
    _____

11

Breaking Out of Trances

Here's the ritual for the scale trance:

1   Wake up, get out of bed, go to the bathroom.

2   Get naked.

3   Stand on the scale.

4   Start a mental tape. Choose one or more of the following:

   ♦   *Why did I eat that yesterday? I am so big and feel so heavy.*

   ♦   *How could that extra ounce of chicken put three pounds on me?*

   ♦   *I'll never be thin enough. I'm hopeless.*

   ♦   *I am so ugly I shouldn't go out of the house.*

   ♦   *Wow! I pigged out all weekend and I'm down two pounds. I ought to pig out all the time.*

   ♦   *I lost a pound. Big deal! At this rate it'll take me until I'm 90 to be the size I want.*

   ♦   *No wonder I don't have a boyfriend/girlfriend/good marriage. Why would anyone in their right mind be attracted to someone this size?*

5   Step off the scale.

6   Feel bad about yourself and repeat these internal messages over and over all through the day.

7   Decide to eat absolutely no pleasurable foods that day, or better yet, plan to avoid eating all day, or just give up and binge.

Clients often ask where the scale is in our office; we don't have one. The reason for this is found in the answers to the following questions: How can weighing be both useful and abusive? What experiences have clients had with weighing at doctors' offices, and what is the best way to handle the weight/scale issue with doctors and others?

⇒   First, body composition is important to use in conjunction with scales to differentiate lean tissue and fat tissue. Scales alone don't accurately reflect calorie usage because lean tissue and fat tissue have a significant difference in the number of calories found in each. You can have a more toned, leaner body that is a different size, and even a different shape, without any change in weight or numbers on the scale. These are reflective of changes in body composition (see Chapter 9).

⇒   Second, eating is often a response to the scale rather than the body's internal signals. No matter what the scale says, it will disrupt a healthy eating pattern or exacerbate an already unhealthy eating pattern. If weight increases, people interpret the increase as a failure to control their eating, so they react by being extremely rigid, by restricting, or by bingeing. If weight remains the same, they are disappointed and interpret the lack of change as a lack of progress, which also results in being extremely rigid, in restricting, or in bingeing. If weight decreases, they often think, *"Yeah, my starving has paid off and my weight's gone down, so I'll continue this restrictive pattern."* Or, the response might be, *"Great! I've made progress. Now I can go eat 'big time' ice cream and a cheeseburger with fries and a shake,"* and so forth. If their weight didn't drop far enough, they restrict further or give up and binge.

⇒ Even though one may realize the pitfalls of weighing illustrated above, many people still want to use the scales regularly. For instance, one of our clients recognized she used the scale to mirror how her mother criticized her as a child; the scale served as another outside evaluation of herself and her body. It was an indicator of being "good enough" or "measuring up." She was uncomfortable or didn't feel "right" or didn't feel as though she was working hard enough unless she had a critical voice chiding her daily .

⇒ Weighing in a physician's office is one of many measurements used to evaluate a person's physical condition. It is not intended as a moral judgment about a person's food consumption. However, it has evolved into sometimes being used as a tool of judgment either by the patient, the physician, or society. Many doctors don't understand the process of intuitive eating. Some of our clients were told by their physicians upon observing their weight to *"Get on the tuna and lettuce and get this taken care of. Just get it off, ace!"* Or to a person undereating, *"Just get some butter in you . . . even better, peanut butter."*

Often, after a visit to the physician or in preparation for a visit, we spend time with clients discussing their feelings and reactions to the nurse and doctor's comments or reactions. This is particularly critical when a client has been tuning into body signals for a significant period of time. Clients are again confronted with evaluations from outside their bodies and by people whom they respect.

Some strategies for diffusing the weight issue in the doctor's office include:

♦ Requesting not to be weighed or asking not to see or be told your weight.

♦ Having a plan for how to respond and a plan for support after the appointment if your weight is revealed. Some possible responses: *"I'm working on this with a nutritionist."* Or, *"I recognize my weight might be causing me problems and I'm addressing that in ways that will help me be less extreme in my eating patterns in the future.*" Or taking this chapter and the chapter on body composition with you and discussing it with him/her.

Ultimately, outside evaluations such as weighing can be deterrents to the intuitive eating process.

Body Part Trance

"When I don't get to exercise I feel my thighs expanding."

"When I eat three meals a day it feels like my stomach expands to the point I'm forced to loosen my belt three notches."

Everybody has parts of their body that they wish were different. And, many of us focus on these parts and treat our whole bodies as if they were only that one part. We try to exercise or starve that part away making the rest of us suffer; we eat only a portion of what our bodies are asking for—and are perfectly miserable with hunger—but try to ignore it. Some of us want to reduce parts and others focus on filling out certain parts, both of which require us to override our intuitive eater. As a result, we feel miserable and usually fail long-term.

This focus on a body part or parts often becomes so intense—even trance-like—the intuitive eater gets ignored or overridden and we spend our time obsessing about the parts we don't like. As a consequence, we miss appreciating the beauty of the integrated whole—all the parts working together, functioning well—even the hated part. For example, if you punish the hated part with exercise, the rest of your body, your mind, and your spirit responds with an inability to focus on anything else or move forward in life. Usually you feel like a failure because the part isn't changing the way you wish it would. Exercise eventually becomes a real pain, difficult, a struggle; you feel tired and irritable—you get very hungry and then struggle with cravings.

No matter which approach to the body parts trance you practice, it keeps you from feeling full and fulfilled. But you can break out of these trances. Begin with the exercises that follow.

Discovering What's Right For You

1   Try skipping one of your routine weigh-ins and notice
how you react. What are the feelings? Do you focus on any
particular part of your body any more or less? Do you eat
differently? Do you exercise differently?

Feelings from not weighing:

_____

_____

_____

Which body parts did you focus on more than others?

_____

_____

How did not weighing affect your eating?

_____

_____

How did not weighing affect your exercise?

_____

_____

2   Continue experimenting with skipping your weigh-ins so
     that there is more and more time between them. How does
     it feel to *think* about that? How does it feel to do it?

Reactions to thinking about weighing less frequently:

_____
_____

Dates you weigh: Feelings about this frequency:

_____   _____

_____   _____

_____   _____

_____   _____

3   When skipping your weigh-ins, do you rely more or less
     on your intuitive eater (body signals)?

Frequency of relying on your intuitive eater:

_____
_____
_____
_____
_____
_____

4   Which body signals do you choose to trust and act on and which do you choose to ignore when you don't weigh?

Body signals	✓ trust	✓ ignore
_____	_____	_____
_____	_____	_____
_____	_____	_____
_____	_____	_____
_____	_____	_____
_____	_____	_____

5   Make a list of all the parts of your body which you wish were different.

Body parts/features you wish were different:

_____

_____

_____

_____

6   Make a list of all the parts of your body that you appreciate just the way they are. (Don't forget skin, nails, hair, face, hands, nose, eyes, lips.)

Body parts/features you like:

_____

_____

_____

_____

7 Keep notes for three days about what and how you decide
to eat through the day. Were your decisions based on your
whole body, your life, your life's purpose, your need for
energy, clarity of thought, or parts of your body? For example: *Am I choosing to eat this way based on signals from
the part of my body I don't like or in response to my intuitive eater's signals? Am I choosing what I know I need to
eat to match my life's journey at this moment?*

Day 1

Foods	Reasons for that choice
_____	_____
_____	_____
_____	_____
_____	_____
_____	_____
_____	_____
_____	_____
_____	_____
_____	_____
_____	_____
_____	_____

Day 2

Foods   Reasons for that choice

_____   _____

_____   _____

_____   _____

_____   _____

_____   _____

_____   _____

_____   _____

_____   _____

_____   _____

_____   _____

_____   _____

_____   _____

Day 3

Foods   Reasons for that choice

_____   _____

_____   _____

_____   _____

_____   _____

_____   _____

_____   _____

_____   _____

_____   _____

_____   _____

_____   _____

_____   _____

_____   _____

chapter

12

Understanding the Impact of Exercise

Most people believe that if they exercise, their metabolic rates will increase, they will burn more calories, and they will lose weight. The truth is not that simple. In fact, people often lower their metabolic rates through exercise and lose muscle weight rather than fat weight. They forget that the type of food, the timing of the food, and the amount of the food they eat is *just* as important.

Using the principles described below, you can make sure you eat and exercise in a manner such that your metabolic rate isn't lowered, and you're not struggling against your body. You may also be able to raise your metabolic rate.

⇒ Calories are fuel that the body burns for energy. Calories are from protein, carbohydrate, fats, and alcohol. Which fuel gets burned during exercise depends on a number of factors: how long and hard you exercise and the amount of carbohydrate you have stored in your body.

⇒ We are always burning some carbohydrate in muscle because it is the body's primary energy source. Approximately one-half of the calories your body burns each day are from carbohydrate. In fact, your body needs carbohydrate *all* the time. Unfortunately, most of us can only store about one-half day's supply of carbohydrate so we need some carbohydrate throughout the day.

⇒ If you don't get enough carbohydrate in your diet, or if you deplete your carbohydrate stores, then your body will break down protein (either from your diet or from your muscle if you haven't eaten enough) and convert it to carbohydrate in the liver to use for energy. This breakdown of muscle protein will lower your metabolic rate because muscle is where most of your calories are burned. When you lose muscle you lessen your ability to burn calories—hence, a lower metabolic rate.

⇒ If you eat more carbohydrate at one meal or snack than your body can store, the extra will get converted to fat. Regrettably, fat *cannot* be converted back to carbohydrate or protein . . . our livers just don't have the enzymes to do that.

⇒ Protein calories are generally not burned for energy unless you haven't eaten enough carbohydrate *and* have also depleted carbohydrate stores. Protein is stored in muscle and is used in other body processes; excess protein is converted to fat.

⇒ Pace and intensity of exercise affect which fuel (protein, carbohydrate, fat, or alcohol) is used. As the intensity of a workout increases, so does the proportion of calories from carbohydrates to total fuel burned. A lower intensity workout tips the balance towards a greater proportion of fat being burned and less carbohydrate which is what most of us struggling with weight want. See the chart that follows:

Fast Pace

2-mile run in 10 minutes

150 carbohydrate calories+50 fat calories = 200 calories

150 carbohydrate calories	50 fat calories

Same person, slower pace

2-mile run in 20 minutes

100 carbohydrate calories+100 fat calories = 200 calories

100 carbohydrate calories	100 fat calories

Intensity of exercise affects appetite. When exercising with greater intensity—which uses a greater proportion of carbohydrate—you will need to eat more carbohydrate and will have an appetite for more carbohydrate after the workout (especially if you have depleted your carbohydrate stores) than when exercising at a lower level of intensity. (However, you can be just as hungry with a low intensity workout if you are depleted of carbohydrate.)

Should you not eat enough carbohydrate and indulge in high intensity workouts, you will break down body proteins and muscle to make carbohydrate. **This is a critical point.** Many people mistakenly believe that if they limit their carbohydrate intake, and then exercise, their body fat will be broken down. What happens, in fact, is that they are lowering their body's capacity to burn fat, and will lower their metabolism. The reason for this is that the body will break down muscle to form carbohydrate. In addition, the muscle breakdown raises stress hormone levels and causes carbohydrate cravings.

When undereating and/or over-exercising, the body and brain chemistry changes initially make people feel powerful, energetic, aggressive, alert and "in control" by releasing dopamine, endorphins and other hormones. Because of these chemical changes, people will often choose to undereat or over-exercise in response to difficult situations in life to produce these alert, powerful, in-control feelings to try to cope. However, over time, the results are all the disadvantages we just discussed—lowered metabolic rate, broken-down muscle, feeling tired, and cravings for carbohydrates.

This chapter offers a very simplistic description of a very complex system of events when exercising. But, by using this knowledge, perhaps you will choose to exercise more moderately, give yourself permission to eat in response to your body's hunger and appetite signals, and raise, or maintain, a high metabolic rate as a result.

Discovering What's Right For You

1   To experience the effect of pace on hunger if you have a
     regular exercise program, increase the intensity for the
     workout and notice any differences in your degree of
     hunger and foods that you think will satisfy your appetite
     best. Again, this is not meant to encourage you to exercise
     faster and become hungrier, it's only a test to experience
     the effects of pace on hunger.

Workout description: _____

Hunger level at regular pace: _____

_____

Hunger level at faster pace: _____

_____

2   If you normally exercise four or five days each week, exper-
     iment with three to four days of no activity and notice what
     your body signals are telling you about how much food
     and the types of food that you need to feel satisfied.

Regular weekly workout   Body signals without regular workout

_____   _____

_____   _____

_____   _____

_____   _____

_____   _____

_____   _____

3   If you don't normally exercise, you may want to exercise moderately for two–three weeks and notice any changes that happen in types and amounts of foods that you want. (Refer to the next three pages before you start this activity.)

Week 1

Describe exercise	Day of week	Length of time for workout
_____	_____	_____
_____	_____	_____
_____	_____	_____
_____	_____	_____

Week 2

Describe exercise	Day of week	Length of time for workout
_____	_____	_____
_____	_____	_____
_____	_____	_____
_____	_____	_____

Week 3

Describe exercise	Day of week	Length of time for workout
_____	_____	_____
_____	_____	_____
_____	_____	_____
_____	_____	_____

For each week, keep notes on the following for each day:

> amount of hunger
> amount of protein
> amount of carbohydrate
> amount of fat
> frequency of cravings/binges

Week 1 Meals

Day 1   Day 2   Day 3   Day 4   Day 5   Day 6   Day 7

For each week, keep notes on the following for each day:

> amount of hunger
> amount of protein
> amount of carbohydrate
> amount of fat
> frequency of cravings/binges

Week 2 Meals

Day 1   Day 2   Day 3   Day 4   Day 5   Day 6   Day 7

For each week, keep notes on the following for each day:

amount of hunger
amount of protein
amount of carbohydrate
amount of fat
frequency of cravings/binges

Week 3 Meals

Day 1   Day 2   Day 3   Day 4   Day 5   Day 6   Day 7

Section Three:

Ending the Struggle

chapter

13 *Progressing Toward Intuitive Eating*

Our experience has shown that people progress through various stages on their paths to eating intuitively. The degree of rigidity and flexibility needed varies with each person's location on the continuum below. More rigidity is required (in the types and amounts of foods, timing of meals and snacks, and frequency of reinforcement) for those in the earlier stages.

Stage 1

Feeling out of control with food (over- and/or under-eating): People at this stage have no relationship between their conscious minds and their physical bodies.

Stage 2

Attempting to feel "in control" by going to extremes with exercise and food.

Stage 3

Trying diet programs: an imposed food structure without regard for internal "locus-of-control." The person follows the imposed structure by rote without responding to body signals.

Stage 4

"Cheating" or sneak eating because diet fails to meet physiological needs. This usually sets up feelings of guilt and shame for not being able to ignore the body's signals such as hunger, lack of energy, moodiness, etc., often resulting in returning to stage 1 or to stage 2.

Stage 5

Starting to recognize and acknowledge the body's signals: for example, noticing that certain eating patterns (amounts, timing, and types of food) produce hunger or satisfaction; or, noticing which foods agree or disagree with the body.

Stage 6

Being apprehensive about these body signals and how to respond to them. As a result, people often regress to earlier stages. (See Chapters 15 and 16 on relapse and resistance.)

Stage 7

Learning to interpret the meaning of each body signal. Exploring whether it is in response to missing something or someone, and afraid to feel something and/or not meeting some basic physical needs. Then reviewing the who, what, when, where of the scenario that may have set up these signals.

Stage 8

Experiencing guided risk-taking: for instance, trying a different quantity of a particular food at a particular meal and noticing the emotional and physical feelings related to this experience. Or, giving yourself pleasure in other ways than with food.

Stage 9

Integrating and applying this learning to food choices and to eating patterns: for example, *"Eating X amount of Y food at Z times makes me feel _____."* Or, *"I notice when I reach for____, I'm really feeling_____."*

Stage 10

Practicing trust in the body's signals and continuing to build on that trust.

Stage 11

Eating intuitively: This is not "perfect" eating, but has the following characteristics: it is individualized, cyclical, and rhythmic; it includes a wide variety of foods; it is free of obsession; it is nourishing, it feels good, and is an essential component of self-care; it enables participation in life rather than feeling imprisoned by food and our bodies. It is knowing that emotions and body signals, both pleasant and unpleasant, are ways that your body and soul let you know how to care for them.

Discovering What's Right For You

1   At which stage are you at this moment?

Currently, I am most often in stage _____.

2   In which stage do you tend to relapse most?

I relapse most often when in stage _____.

3   In which stage have you spent the most time over the past
     week, the past month, the past year?

The past week I have been mostly in stage _____.

The past month I have been mostly in stage _____.

The past year I have been mostly in stage _____.

chapter

14 *Using Food Journals To Avoid Punishment*

Many people's experiences with food records have been quite demoralizing and humiliating: a homework assignment to be turned in to the teacher, a confession of guilt to a parent, or a self-punishment tool.

A client, reluctantly, decided to journal her food for a week to help her have a clearer picture of "good" food days and "bad" food days. In the past, she had kept food records frequently and turned them in to be judged as good or bad.

When she returned with her journal, we greeted her with *"What did you notice about food from keeping these journals?"* We and she began to notice fewer servings of complex carbohydrate for 2–3 days preceding the "bad" day (the one containing a milkshake and four cookies). Also, she noticed breakfast that day was only cottage cheese and pineapple, lunch a broth-based soup.

Based on these discoveries, she realized she was meeting her carbohydrate needs with readily-available and easily digested carbohydrate foods such as shakes and cookies, possibly as a result of two days of inadequate complex carbohydrate intake. (See Chapter 6.)

Because of this experience of using her journals to explore and learn, her face brightened as she exclaimed, *"You don't know how I have dreaded showing you these records, and now I feel so freed!"*

What strikes us as surprising is how rarely food journals have been used as tools for exploration and education.

If she had come in the next week without increasing carbohydrates, the food journal would, again, serve as a tool to explore the reasons she avoided getting enough carbohydrate-rich food.

Was she experiencing discomfort, bloating, or fullness from having more carbohydrate or certain types of carbohydrates?

Was it unavailable—no time for the grocery store?

Was she fearful of weight gain?

In other words, using a person's food journal can help get past what many people see as unmotivated, lazy, and "non-compliant" behavior. However, for some people, given their history with food, food-journaling is not a good idea. For example: the person who continues to punish herself with the journal and is unable to shift to an exploring, deciphering mode, or people who use food records as a structure and standard that must be followed as opposed to a non-judgmental tool to gain insight and explore their bodies and food.

So, as with every part of the process toward intuitive eating, whether, and how, journals are used needs to be based on individual needs.

Discovering What's Right For You

1   Have you used food journals before? What was your experience? How did it feel? Did it help?

Describe your past experiences with food journals.

_____

_____

_____

_____

_____

2   Recall and record what you ate and drank yesterday and today. Review your list and notice what feelings and thoughts come to mind.

Day 1	Day 2
_____	_____
_____	_____
_____	_____
_____	_____
_____	_____
_____	_____
_____	_____
_____	_____
_____	_____
_____	_____
_____	_____
_____	_____

As you look at the list, describe your thoughts and feelings.

3   From activity number two, do you recognize any patterns
     about food and eating that you weren't aware of?

Describe any patterns you see.

_____

_____

_____

_____

chapter

15 *Relapsing Into Old Patterns*

First, it is important to realize that relapse is normal and can happen at every point on the journey. It is very rare that anyone progresses smoothly through uncovering their intuitive eater without relapse.

Second, relapse is often a normal body's response to physical choices and/or emotional situations and does not mean failing. For instance, overeating can be the result of a physiological set-up: demands placed on the body. An earlier decision or situation could result in the body failing to receive the amounts, types, textures, etc. of foods it needs to be in balance and well-fueled. (See Chapter 5.)

For example, George normally eats a sandwich, chips, vegetables, and juice for lunch to satisfy his taste, texture, and nutrient needs. But one day there isn't time to eat, so instead of his usual, he eats pretzels and juice from the vending machine. That evening, he gets a fast-food double cheeseburger, and extra-large order of french fries, and a large milk shake. Two hours later, he dives into a carton of ice cream. In contrast, his more typical dinner might be pork chops, a cup of mashed potatoes, salad, a roll or two, and later, some cookies for dessert.

George's lunch altered his body and brain chemistry such that there was a physiological drive to seek out certain kinds of foods and to overeat in an attempt to bring the body back into balance. (See Chapter 6.)

The set-up for relapse could also be emotional. (See Chapter 4.) Feelings change the body and brain chemistry and, in turn, create a desire or craving for certain kinds of foods in order to bring the body back into balance. For example, feelings of anxiety, anger, happiness, sadness, excitement, etc. change body and brain biochemistry, which in turn affect appetite. Understanding this allows you to *use* relapses to help you learn how your body reacts to physical and emotional set-ups.

Rather than isolated situations, as in George's case, sometimes the set-ups are a repeated pattern of circumstances. Maggie gets up at 5:00 a.m. She fixes breakfast and lunch for her husband and kids, takes the kids to school, goes to work, and leaves work in time to pick up the kids. Her next three hours are spent shuttling the children from one activity and appointment to another. Then Maggie rushes home to prepare dinner and feed the family in shifts, according to their individual schedules. Next she does some household chores. After listening to the kids talk about their day and helping them finish their homework, she puts them to bed. At this point in her day she feels drained, impatient, and frustrated because there is so much more she feels she should be doing. She dreads the remainder of the week, which she knows will only bring more of the hectic exhaustion. On particularly exasperating days, when the house is finally quiet, she collapses into an easy chair and gives herself a reward—the soothing, sweet coolness of frozen yogurt paired with soft, chewy brownies.

We, as nutritionists, help clients who have "relapsed" take a step back for a more objective, less emotional, less critical view of the eating behavior. We do this by helping clients evaluate whether or not their physical needs for carbohydrate, protein and fat were met; whether or not their prior meals and snacks were satisfying, or if there is any sense of deprivation prior to the "out-of-control" eating episode. If they over-ate simply as a coping tool for some emotional trigger, like Maggie in our example, we suggest they explore developing other coping tools (often with the help of a counselor or other professional) rather than spend valuable time and emotional energy berating themselves about their food choices.

Distancing yourself emotionally and reviewing the set-ups to the problem eating situation will enable you to discover what can be done differently the next time. This can dilute the more typical, disabling reactions of feeling remorse, shame, failure, and self-loathing. The less critical, more problem-solving approach creates a sense of power, which alters body and brain chemistry to actually diminish food cravings.

Discovering What's Right For You

1   Review a past eating situation that you are unhappy about
    or wish that you had handled differently.

List some of the possible physiological reasons for this relapse.
(You may want to review Chapters 5 and 6 as you think about it.)

_____

_____

_____

_____

List any possible emotional cues that might have played a role.
(You may want to review Chapter 4 to help with this.)

_____

_____

_____

_____

Describe how you responded to the relapse. Some examples might be:

I decided not to eat the next meal

I signed up for a new diet program

I told myself what a lazy failure I was

I cried and didn't want to leave the house

_____

_____

_____

_____

Reviewing the above notes from your relapse, describe how you might try to prevent a similar situation in the future.

_____

_____

_____

_____

Describe your typical reaction to a relapse.

_____

_____

_____

_____

2   When you experience your next relapse, come back to this chapter and try to work #1 rather than repeat your usual relapse. Keep notes about how responding differently to a relapse feels.

Autobiography In Five Short Chapters

by Portia Nelson

I

I walk down the street.
>There is a deep hole in the sidewalk.
>I fall in.
>I am lost . . . I am helpless.
>It isn't my fault.
It takes forever to find a way out.

II

I walk down the same street.
>There is a deep hole in the sidewalk.
>I pretend I don't see it.
>I fall in again.
I can't believe I am in the same place.
>But, it isn't my fault.
It still takes a long time to get out.

III

I walk down the same street.
>There is a deep hole in the sidewalk.
>I see it is there.
>I still fall in . . . it's a habit.
>my eyes are open.
>>I know where I am.
>It is my fault.
I get out immediately.

IV

I walk down the same street.
>There is a deep hole in the sidewalk.
I walk around it.

V

I walk down another street.

16 *Resisting and Fear of Success*

Your dream comes true! You have a body that you like and you eat the way you've always wanted.

How would you feel?

What would you do?

What would your body be like?

Most people *expect* their reaction to be one of relief, excitement, contentment and peace.

But, most of our clients discover that underneath this fantasy are lots of expectations and fears, in fact, so many, that on an unconscious level they make sure they never actually achieve their dream so they can avoid facing these fears.

Each of us has expectations of who we would be if we were at our ideal weight and were at peace with food. Rarely, however, do we pull up these expectations from the unconscious and look at them. When we do, it is usually quite a surprise. People usually recognize that there is logic behind their sabotage, lack of willpower, and resistances.

"Everything I don't like in myself at my current size would be different if I could just lose weight" is many people's unconscious expectation. Think about it, to live up to *that* sounds *so* impossible and scary, who *wouldn't* make sure they never get there?

All of us have a particular image of who or what it means to be an ideal size—no matter how unrealistic it may be—and rarely do we even recognize that we act based on these images.

Some examples from our clients:

"If I am lean and trim and healthy, I would have to act like a stereotypical superficial, ditzy, shallow, yuppie."

"If I am at ideal weight, I will never be able to eat any foods just for pleasure."

"If I am at ideal weight, I will never be able to skip a workout."

"If I'm happy with my looks, I must feel confident, successful, and attractive all the time."

"If I'm at a normal weight, people will notice my body everywhere I go and comment on my appearance."

"If I achieve my goal weight, I'll have to cope with others wanting me sexually and I don't know how to protect myself."

"If I am naturally introverted, as soon as I am happy with my weight, I must be an outgoing party animal."

"I enjoy having a messy home and hate to clean, yet if I stop struggling with food I have to have a clean, minimalist, abstract metal and white pristine home."

"If I am happy with my weight, I won't have anything to struggle with, worry about, etc. What would I do with all the time left that I used to spend thinking about food?"

There are some really good reasons people don't achieve their goal: one is fear—usually totally unknown to them on a conscious level. This constant, underlying fear and anxiety changes body biochemistry and sets up a physiological drive for food—specific foods which can alter hormones and bring comfort. (See Chapters 4-6.) This constant state of anxiety creates feelings of hopelessness about ever reaching this goal and shame about not having enough will-power when the root is hidden fears.

Another reason for not achieving your goal is more immediate: As we mentioned in Chapter 5, as you begin to eat to match your physical needs, you will not be covering up your emotional needs. This may allow feelings that have been suppressed to surface or you may be more sensitive to discomfort in your current situation. Don't be surprised if you want to go back to undereating or overeating as a way to get relief. This can be an opportunity to use some of the supportive ideas in Chapter 23 to handle the discomfort.

Instead of criticizing, judging, and shaming yourself, recognize you are often just scared. And, often, when we look at the hidden fears, we recognize that some are humorous and not real and others can be handled by learning specific techniques for coping. Having the hidden become known gives you a feeling of power and hopeful-ness.

The belief system is: *"I'm required to be or do things that I don't like or don't know how to do if I lose weight."* **Not true.** The reality: *"I can choose to enjoy solitude whatever my weight. I can choose to have a clean or messy house whatever my weight, etc."*

In working with our clients, we can't remember a time when their resistance didn't tell us something that we and they needed to know. It always comes back to the unconscious fears that we just discussed. All the support groups, diet programs, plans, resolutions and contracts cannot make peace happen with food and your body in the long term unless these fears and resistances are understood. We've explained physical and emotional situations that affect food desires in Chapters 4 and 5. This is different. This is about under-standing that some part of you doesn't feel able to deal with what you believe will be expected of you when you are at peace with your weight.

Often, clients label these unconscious fears and beliefs as their "rebel." On the surface, it's:

> *"I'm resisting."*
>
> *"I'm rebelling."*
>
> *"I know what to eat, I just don't do it."*
>
> *"I commit to eating low-fat, but eat donuts in response."*
>
> *"I'm not motivated, I'm too lazy, I just don't have the willpower."*
>
> *"Why can't I do this? I just can't get myself to do* _____.*"*

But underneath the "rebel" is a loving, supportive protector that believes all the unconscious fears and beliefs and makes sure you don't succeed so you won't have the pain of what it believes will happen when you do. The more you ignore it or try to fight it, the more intense and rebellious it becomes. The intent of the rebel is always loving, caring and protective, but how it acts is often hurtful and its beliefs about what must happen if you stop struggling with food are, as we just discussed, often humorous, not always logical, and can be changed, worked with, and released.

For example, the person who resists and rebels against exercise may:

1 have only experienced pain and discomfort while exercising

2 believe they must spend hours exercising to "get rewards"

3 fear ridicule from thinner, more athletic people

4 feel embarrassed about how they look or their lack of coordination. In other words, past experience says exercising causes pain in some way. The rebel is trying to protect them from that pain

5   recognize that if they add exercise to their current food
plan, they will be successful in losing weight. And if
they are successful, then . . . (as listed on page 104)

Listen to your rebel. What is it trying to tell you under its ac-
tions, under its resistance? What is the fear that it is trying to protect you from?

Once you really know the fears and beliefs that your "rebel" is
acting out, you can then acknowledge and recognize all the pain and
discomfort your rebel is trying to protect you from. This new information can then be used as a base to address and problem-solve the
unconscious concerns, pain, and fear.

Sometimes, that means you build around it. For example: if
exhaustion from exercise is the pain or fear, and the rebel is trying
to protect you from this, look for ways that you can exercise and not
have to experience the exhaustion. Maybe doing the activity with
less intensity, or making sure you're eating enough to fuel your activity, or doing fewer other activities so you are less tired and have
more time to enjoy your exercise or getting more sleep so you're not
as tired.

If you feel stupid when exercising, ask what stupid means—
awkward, embarrassed that you're having to do this, uncoordi-
nated—then based on what the answers are, come up with some options that address the feeling.

Maybe find another location to exercise that doesn't feel as uncomfortable, find another time when fewer people would be around,
experiment with other, more comfortable activities that require less
coordination, and so on.

Over time, as you practice listening and responding to your
rebel's concerns, you'll see what a valuable tool your resistance is
and instead of hating yourself for having a rebel you'll be able to
interpret resistance as fears and beliefs you don't know about yet.

Discovering What's Right For You

1   What are your belief systems? *"If I were thin, how would I feel? What would I think? What would I have to do?"*

If I were comfortable with my body size and how I was eating, then:

_____

_____

_____

_____

_____

2   Take each one of the answers in #1 and identify which ones you're scared about or feel you don't have the tools to do, or don't fit with who you think you *really* are or want to be.

I'm scared of or don't really want which of the above:

_____

_____

_____

_____

_____

3   Which of these *at this point* are logical consequences of being your desired weight or eating differently? Which of these are not required consequences?

   Circle those listed in #1 that you feel are logical consequences. Put an "x" next to those that are not required consequences.

4   Choose one of the consequences or fears that you would like to develop more confidence about, or have less fear about. Read about or seek professional guidance on how to address it and ease the fear of living without your struggle with food.

   Put a star next to the one you would like to currently face.

5   List one area of your struggle with food that you seem to have the most resistance to. Check with your "rebel." It is trying to tell you something about your fears and beliefs that you need to know. *"If I accomplish this, what am I afraid will happen that I won't like or that would be scary?"* Then, come up with one way you can start to address the fears it tells you about.

   _____
   _____
   _____
   _____
   _____

chapter

17

Sneak Eating

Ah! Nobody's home. What a relief. Take advantage of this time to eat . . . foods you don't want anybody to know you eat . . . in volumes you don't want anybody to know you want. Maybe even throw it up but nobody will know. Feel the freedom. Feel the exhilaration. Feel the relief. Then, feel the fear, the shame, the humiliation, the self-loathing.

Sneak eating is an indicator, a symbol of some real needs that we are usually afraid to admit we have, afraid that we aren't supposed to have, and afraid that we don't know any other way of addressing. It's usually a time when we can be the "real me" with all our wants and desires. It is a time when you don't have to pretend to be competent, confidant, mature, able to handle anything, and have no needs. It is a time to be totally self-centered, when you don't have to take care of anyone else and can focus totally on yourself.

Every healthy human needs time to be who they really are, have needs and wants, satisfy those needs and wants, and focus solely on themselves. Ironically, most of us were taught these healthy human desires were selfish, impolite, unimportant, and shameful. So, most of us try to ignore and pretend we don't feel the deep longing that is calling us to this solitude, reflection, and self-satisfaction.

Instead, we hide, lie, and make excuses about our need for alone time. We pretend we don't need or want pleasure and override it in all areas of our life. We substitute food for pleasures in life. We fight food. We try to force ourselves not to eat, *especially* not sneak eat. And, we punish and criticize ourselves for not being able to stop.

So, recognize that sneak eating is *not* about you having shameful desires that cannot be controlled. Instead, sneak eating indicates you have healthy, natural, human longings that you were not taught how to address. If sneak eating is a real problem for you, you may want to spend more time reading and doing the activities in the next chapter on pleasure.

18

Hunger for Pleasure

What are you truly hungry for in life? What is your greatest longing? We're not talking about what you wish for your children or what you wish for your spouse. Focus on you. What is *your* greatest longing? Not considering the question *"What am I truly hungry for in life?"* is at the base of most people's struggle with food. *"What would give me the **most** pleasure and satisfaction?"* If we are willing to face that question and act on it, we often struggle less with weight and food.

It is human and healthy to want pleasure. Also, it is healthy to make sure you get pleasure. But for most people, giving themselves pleasure is guilt-ridden, selfish, something to hide and often accompanied by a full dose of fear. Because of the guilt and fear, most of us override this pleasure-seeking instinct and pretend we can live without it. The more we daily deprive ourselves of pleasure the more our desire for it intensifies. And, often, the more our need for pleasure in every area of life is ignored, the more unruly and unmanageable food becomes.

Food is a very popular substitute for the lack of pleasure in broader and deeper areas of our life. We all have certain foods that provide pleasure—usually those we restrict our intake of. Food is convenient, often one of the most easily accessible sources of pleasure. Eating can be done alone—a plus, since giving in to our need for pleasure is often so guilt-ridden.

And, using food for pleasure, *especially* if done alone, doesn't cause as much conflict as other pleasurable things we might desire, like changing jobs to something we really enjoy, moving to a part of the country we love, doing activities that the rest of the family doesn't enjoy, etc. The feeling of pleasure, whether from food, art, dance, friends, meditation, or anything else changes the body's hormonal balance. (See Chapters 4 and 6)

So, to relieve pain and feel pleasure, food is not the only option. All pleasure, whether from food or not, causes changes in endorphin levels. And eating a balance of carbohydrates, fats, proteins, textures, flavors, temperatures, and density of food—avoiding both chronic hunger and overeating—bring even more pleasure, due to its changes in endorphin levels in the brain and body.

How many subtle ways do you override your pleasure on a daily basis?

- ◆ Going to the bathroom when you need to rather than holding it until you finish your duties.
- ◆ Eating meals when you are truly hungry.
- ◆ Choosing foods that satisfy you.
- ◆ Going to bed when you are sleepy.
- ◆ Choosing to say no to an invitation with people you don't enjoy being with.
- ◆ Working at a job you truly enjoy.
- ◆ Resting when you are tired.
- ◆ Asking for attention or a hug when you need reassurance.
- ◆ Wearing clothes and shoes that aren't uncomfortable or binding.

- Making love when and how you most enjoy it.
- Taking time to play.

These are just a few of the many opportunities we have daily to give ourselves pleasure. But, most of us override our need for pleasure in every arena of life: our relationships, our food, our jobs, our balance of time spent working and playing, etc. And it is often done out of fear.

> *"What will people think?"*
> *"I'll be a bad parent if I do things for **my** pleasure."*
> *"I don't deserve pleasure."*
> *"I don't have time."*
> *"I'll be out of control and lose all sense of responsibility."*

How do you go about satisfying your hunger for pleasure and overcoming your fears and guilt about your need for pleasure? Oddly enough, most of us have worked so hard at not giving ourselves pleasure that we actually have linked pleasure with some of our most painful situations to try to make them easier to bear (for example, a sense of pleasure when we feel hungry after we've restricted our food intake). We have come to associate the pain of hunger with pleasure.

Pleasure in every arena in life is required for you to be whole and healthy. You can learn to honor your own instincts about what is pleasurable for you and learn to balance what gives you pleasure with your responsibilities for self-care, family, school and community.

Discovering What's Right For You

1   Take an inventory of you and your pleasure. Make a list of
     those things you do that *don't* bring you pleasure and
     make a list of those things that *do* bring you pleasure.
     Look for the subtle things as well as the more obvious.
     Choose one item that you would like to try to do more
     frequently.

Things I enjoy   Things I don't get pleasure from

_____   _____

_____   _____

_____   _____

_____   _____

_____   _____

Put a ✓ next to the one you would like to focus on more often in your life.

2   Write down the one you would like to try to add to your
     life. Then, explore it by filling in the blank with as many
     fears and possible bad outcomes as you can think of. *"If I
     do this, then* _____ *."* For
     example: *"If I do this, then: my spouse will get mad, my
     friends will make fun of me, I'll go out of control, I'll lose
     my job, I'll feel embarrassed and ashamed, etc."* Try to fill
     a page with fears and guilt. This exercise helps us under-
     stand that withholding pleasure from yourself in some
     ways protects you from having to face fear and guilt but
     also makes most people feel deprived, restricted, trapped,
     or angry.

When you finish your list, review it. Usually, many of the fears on the list are ones that we designed as kids without much logic or reality to them when we look at them as adults. Those that do have some validity we can often discuss and create ways to minimize their impact. For example, you're afraid your spouse will get mad. Maybe you could share that you'd like to do this and are concerned he or she will be angry with you; the two of you might brainstorm some ways to balance both of your needs. Often, however, just being really honest and verbalizing the fears is sufficient to release enough of the resistance and fear that you can go ahead and do it.

How will I make this less scary to try?

_____
_____
_____
_____

3   List some ways that you might have fun on a regular basis. Adults in our society have very few options to play if we follow our cultural norms: eating out; getting together for drinks; inviting people over for dinner. These are *the* most common outlets for us as adults to play and they all involve food. What are other ways you could incorporate more fun/pleasure and some ways that don't involve food? Most of us allow ourselves a long weekend or a vacation once a year but humans need pleasure daily.

Fun without food:

_____
_____
_____

4   Notice if you ever eat and then get angry at yourself for doing it. These are usually times when you did some type of pleasure override and are substituting food for what you really wanted. Write a brief paragraph about the experience and see if you can identify what pleasure you wanted. Many times, it is something like a hug or someone to listen to you.

What pleasure did you substitute food for?:

_____
_____
_____
_____
_____

5   Write down a list of foods, snacks and/or meals you might enjoy eating. Or, write down the most satisfying, pleasurable food that you can imagine. This may change from day to day, week to week or season to season.

List some pleasurable foods you rarely allow yourself to have:

_____   _____
_____   _____
_____   _____
_____   _____

6   Experiment by including a pleasurable food that you usu-
     ally try to avoid—*without using it as a substitute for plea-
     sure you're missing somewhere else.* Most of us who strug-
     gle with allowing ourselves pleasure have difficulty giving
     ourselves permission to include pleasurable foods into our
     regular pattern of eating without guilt and fear.

     Yet if we do this in balance with other healthy foods the
     emotional charge that builds up around these pleasurable
     foods often minimizes. It is very rewarding to begin the
     process of separating your longing and hunger for plea-
     sure from pleasurable foods. This separation allows you to
     enjoy both and not have to overuse food to make up for a
     lack somewhere else. And, by working on these steps, you
     will begin to do this.

     Choose one pleasurable food and include it as part of a meal this next week.
     Describe the experience:

     _____

     _____

     _____

     _____

7 Consider pleasure as you decide what to eat at meals. Think about what textures, what temperatures, what taste combinations would sound satisfying and pleasurable as you decide what to eat. Eating something cold, creamy, and sweet when you are really wanting something warm, crunchy and salty—or vice-versa— is usually unsatisfying and often is a setup to overeat.

Describe sensations and feelings before, during, and after a meal where your pleasure was not considered:

_____

_____

_____

Describe sensations and feelings as above, when you chose your meal based on pleasure:

_____

_____

_____

chapter

19

Surviving the Holidays

Surprise! This is *not* one more story full of tips about what you should and shouldn't do with food during the holidays. Beginning with Halloween and continuing through New Years (and perhaps even Valentines and Easter) holiday tips and advice will abound in all kinds of women's and health and cooking magazines, T.V. shows and newspapers right along with recipes for the lowest fat and highest fat dinners and party foods. Tips for planning ahead to eat *just* what you think you should, not depriving yourself, drinking diet sodas between alcoholic beverages, avoiding the little quiches and opting for the cherry tomatoes and yogurt dip, not going to a party hungry, and dealing with food gifts—all may help. But, they may also accentuate the problems of holiday eating and divert you from a solution for a deeper struggle, a struggle which many men and women wage, especially during November and December.

This chapter is about what's at the root of our struggle with food during the holidays. Food and alcohol are primary players during this season because they alter emotions. In most cases we set ourselves up, with society's help, for a "no-win" conflict around food. You show up for a party or even just go to work and are expected to join in, be a part of the crowd and the mood, and eat whatever is there. If you *don't* eat, you feel "righteous" or "right" but feel as if you don't fit in—uncomfortable, guilty. If you *do* eat what's offered, you fit in; your colleagues feel comfortable, they have company. You, though, may feel guilty because you're not doing what you "ought." Thus, the "no-win" conflict of the holidays.

During the holidays, most of us rarely have a sense of success with what we choose to eat. This holiday conflict with food is often a metaphor for another holiday conflict: that of participating in holiday rituals and activities because you are *expected* to do so by family, friends, and co-workers versus participating in rituals because you *want* to. "Doing the expected" often leaves us feeling frustrated, drained, inadequate, powerless, angry, empty, and un-nurtured. In other words, fulfilling these obligations rarely "feeds" us. So, we feed ourselves with food. In addition, we do what is expected, believing it will provide us with warm, fuzzy, close connections with family and friends. When we don't feel these close connections, we use food to create the "warm fuzzies." Food does this by changing our brain chemistry, which alters our moods, as we've discussed. In contrast, choosing to be involved with people we truly enjoy and in activities which we truly *want* to do, nurtures, satisfies, and actually "feeds" us. Like eating food, doing things you enjoy creates changes in brain chemistry and affects moods.

A Word About Alcohol

Drinking alcohol, perhaps in even a more profound way than eating, alters brain chemistry and feelings as well. Therefore, it, too, is often "used" more during the holidays when stress is high and feelings of loneliness are accentuated. Also, alcohol makes the struggle with food even harder because it interferes with the liver's ability to process carbohydrates and proteins so these foods are not as available to balance brain chemistry.

Therefore, the day after drinking alcohol, people often have an appetite for a lot more sweets and starches or high fat, protein-rich foods.

Let's look at what you can do:

⇒ Recognize that your struggle with food and eating often has at its root some conflict about doing what you *want* to do versus what you *think others expect* you to do; trying to get "fed" by doing what you *should* do—not just with food but with the whole holiday season. We may want the close, warm contacts and intimate sharing with people that we have been taught to expect during this time of year but we often don't feel these. This sets up the desire to eat to create these sensations— biochemically, as a substitute.

⇒ You might want to identify situations where you struggle with what you want to do and what you think others expect you to do. If necessary, seek professional guidance to help you partici- pate in a way that will actually "feed" you because of what you do and who you do it with. This will deal with the root of your struggle with food.

⇒ If you notice that you are feeling angry at yourself about your food choices and/or quantities through the holidays, try to look past the food and see if you can identify the "I want" versus the "I'm expected" conflict. Feeling angry at yourself about your eating only keeps you stuck—wanting to eat more to attempt to change your brain chemistry to mask the anger which, in turn, makes you feel more anger at yourself, and the cycle continues.

⇒ Recognize that eating what your body needs to be well-fueled throughout the day provides a foundation to minimize cravings and out-of-control eating at parties, etc. because it balances brain chemistry.

Discovering What's Right For You

1   List the holiday situations and rituals that truly give you pleasure. While doing this, you will probably be able to create a list of situations that don't give you pleasure, as well.

Pleasurable holiday activities   Not pleasurable

_____   _____
_____   _____
_____   _____
_____   _____
_____   _____
_____   _____

2   Identify which of the above you do because you want to versus those you do because you're "expected" to.

Place a ✔ next to those you do because you want to.

3   As you attend different holiday events, make notes about how you felt about your eating—food choices, quantity, etc. noting if you see any patterns between your eating and the "if you wanted to" versus "were expected to" attend.

_____
_____
_____
_____
_____

20 *Anticipating Change*

Paulette had a routine during the school year: After she dropped off the kids, she went to the park for a workout, home for a relaxing shower and peaceful breakfast. She then actually had time to do something fun or creative. Later, she was able to get a lunch that really satisfied her—just the right tastes, temperature, textures, colors, etc.—all that she was in the mood for. This allowed her to feel good, with energy for the afternoon chores and evening family time.

But when school was out for the summer, she didn't go exercise because she couldn't leave the kids at home alone. Breakfast was on the run. Lunch was "kid's food" in between feeding the kids all morning. She found herself eating all the different foods—popsicles, chips, etc.—that she bought for their summer treats. By the end of the day, she was exhausted, uncentered, and only wanted to get dinner at the drive-through.

Any change or transition, no matter how big or small, affects how you take care of yourself. Therefore, you can anticipate having to make some shifts in your self-care routines. Rather than "falling" into a pattern and then having to climb back out of that pattern as a result of the transition, you may want to think in advance how you want to create new patterns, habits, and routines. This helps you deal with any transition with the greatest ease. It's important to consider how you want to feel, what your ideal day would be with exercise and food, and some possible ways to organize your day and activities to achieve this. *Exploring* is a key word to the transition process, recognizing that you're going to need to try some different approaches to find the best new pattern for you.

In other words, you're going to try some things that do not work; this is normal and to be expected. If it's summer, think about the transition involved in kids getting out of school, or going on vacation, or coming back after vacation to work. Think about all the changes that these *normal* transitions affect in your exercise routine, sleep/wake cycle, water/fluid intake, meal patterns, types of food, logistics of getting food, how food is prepared, *and* as a result, how it makes you feel.

If you can anticipate changes and choose to plan for the greatest enjoyment, you'll avoid the guilt and discomfort that often follows falling into eating and exercise patterns that don't make you feel good.

Some examples of transitions that people overlook, but which often affect eating patterns, are:

- moving (different food sources, new schedules, new kitchen arrangement, restaurants)
- travel/vacations
- weekdays to weekends (more/less time, schedules vary)
- home to college to working world
- seasonal change (different availability of food, wanting different textures, flavors, heartiness, lightness)
- marriage/divorce
- new roommates
- celebrations/holidays
- work shift change
- new baby
- house guests/relatives

Discovering What's Right For You

1   Make a list of transitions in your life that are likely to leave you more vulnerable to your old patterns.

   List transitions you are going through currently or anticipate happening in the next several weeks.

   _____
   _____
   _____
   _____
   _____
   _____
   _____
   _____
   _____
   _____

2   Then make a list of precautions that you can take in the face of these transitions.

   What disruptions or difficulties with self-care are you experiencing or can you anticipate during this transition? Explore some ways you can prevent them.

   _____
   _____
   _____
   _____
   _____
   _____

chapter

21

Practicing
at
Mealtime

*Amy recounted her most satisfying recent meal: the bril-
liant saffron yellow of the chilled orange juice in the glisten-
ing, crystal clear pitcher; the royal blue plates set on lime
green place mats with crisp red napkins; the aroma of warm-
ing maple syrup and pancakes floating in the air; the delight-
ful contrast of the fresh, firm, tart strawberries with the
warm, soft sweetness of the pancakes and syrup; and the
soothing murmur of surrounding family and friends.*

There's more to eating than following rules. Intuitive eating
requires that you recognize what provides pleasure and satisfaction.
This ensures that you nourish the body, mind, *and* soul.

Most of us have forgotten how to do this. To get back in touch
with being satisfied when you eat, we suggest taking time at some of
your meals to try some of the following tools for intuitive eating.
Certainly, it is impractical and unrealistic to expect yourself to do all
of these at every meal every day. The idea is to be aware of how these
tools impact how you feel about yourself and how you feed yourself
and incorporate whichever ones are useful as often as possible.

⇒ Consider the colors, textures, temperatures, flavors, aroma, and shapes of the different foods when choosing your meal. A variety of these within a meal leads to a deeper level of satisfaction.

⇒ Ask yourself how hungry you are for this type of meal. Ask yourself how much you want.

⇒ Breathe deeply and mentally scan your body. Notice how ready it is for the food you've chosen.

⇒ Arrange food on a plate—even if it's take-out. Allow yourself to anticipate the flavors, textures, etc. of the food.

⇒ Pause to notice and enjoy the aromas.

⇒ Create a pleasant environment for eating—set up a quiet, relaxed mood by getting away from irritating noises, fast or loud music, TV, phones; think about the color of your plate, the place mat, etc.

⇒ Consider the time, energy and thought that went into this meal: the growing, harvesting, and transporting; the planning of the meal; the preparing of the meal. Think about all of this human and natural energy which will be incorporated into your being.

⇒ With the first bite, notice the sensations, such as the burst of *flavors* and how they change as you chew; next, notice the *textures* and how they change as you chew; then, notice the *sounds* as you chew and swallow.

⇒ Ask yourself:

Is it more satisfying to chew for a short time or longer?

Do the size of the bites make a difference?

Are there particular textures or flavors that are more appealing or is it the combination of these?

Do you get more satisfaction from chewing or swallowing?

As you begin to finish your meal, check your hunger and satisfaction. Is there anything missing that will seal your sense of satisfaction—for example, taking another bite, something to drink, something sweet or sour, crunchy, smooth, cold, or warm?

If this meal didn't satisfy, make sure you attempt to incorporate what was missing into another meal or snack within the next day or two.

We find the more clearly people can identify what satisfies them, the less time they spend thinking about food. They experience less overeating. In addition, they actually start enjoying their meals!

chapter

22

*Evolving
into a
New Lifestyle*

How many times have you said, *"I'm going to change my lifestyle. It's time to get on a new program, especially with the way I eat?"* Doesn't it feel good to start fresh? But it seems you can't sustain it and need to keep starting over. Why?

The stock answer is: the new lifestyle is not individualized. But, it is so much more than that. In fact, the program you try to change to may be physiologically correct but rarely does it address the many different elements that make up your lifestyle:

- ◆ moods
- ◆ cycles
- ◆ seasons
- ◆ schedules
- ◆ transitions
- ◆ activity levels
- ◆ social situations
- ◆ likes and dislikes
- ◆ past experiences
- ◆ level of trust

and the most important element—discovery about *what is right for you* about each of these elements.

For instance, a client chooses to limit fat and is successful for a couple of months, then just quits. Why? Could it be because this lifestyle change didn't consider all these elements of life that affect how he/she eats and breathes and moves? Some of these elements are in our control to change, others we don't even know about to try to change or don't know how to change, and some we just can't control or change.

A new program to change your lifestyle rarely addresses all your changing physiological needs and all your changing emotional needs. *One critical factor is when people begin to eat well they become more aware of their feelings*—which can be painful and uncomfortable. These feelings often cause people to revert back to their old patterns.

Starting a new lifestyle is more accurately described as *evolving* into a new lifestyle—exploring and experimenting with each element that affects it. Some examples: discovering how your mental state affects your cravings; how your exercise affects your cravings; which moods affect food choices and amounts; how much time you have available to prepare and think about food; how taste, texture, flavor, temperature, and volume affect your satisfaction, etc.

Therefore, plan to evolve into a new lifestyle. Allow for self-discovery about all the little elements which will make up your personal lifestyle—and eating style; don't force yourself into a "program."

Discovering What's Right For You

1   Create your ideal day incorporating as many details as you can think of that would make eating pleasurable and satisfying. Review, in this chapter, the list of different elements as you create your ideal day.

List details that would make eating pleasurable and satisfying:

_____

_____

_____

_____

_____

_____

_____

_____

_____

_____

_____

_____

chapter

23

Support and Other Resources

You are the ultimate authority on what is best for you. This book has helped you recognize that you have an intuitive system available to discern or determine what techniques work best for tuning in to your needs; what food, timing, meals, etc. are the best match for you. But, we all need support and teachers to introduce us to new ideas or help guide us or help us reflect on our experiences. We strongly recommend finding a person, group or program that works with a style that will allow you to be more and more confident in exploring and using your own intuitive system; that can either point to new pathways to discovering your body's intuitive messages and/or reinforce and strengthen the systems that already work for you.

Just because you find a nutritionist, counselor, massage therapist, dance teacher—whoever works in this area, or however good their intent—doesn't mean that this person necessarily is the best match for you. You may need different *kinds* and *styles* of support at different times and stages of your exploration. For some people, this may mean following a path of doing body work, dance, or movement; others may need a therapist, others a spiritual counselor.

The helper, program or professional you go to should use terms like *"I suggest," "You might try," "Experiment with," "Listen to," "Explore."* Their suggestions will be based not only on facts, but also on their, and your, personal experience. They will always encourage you to reflect and use your intuitive system to guide you. You should also feel safe with this person.

After people begin eating and moving in ways that nurture their bodies and souls, they are far more "open" to feeling things they have never felt, or at least never felt with the intensity that they may now feel them. We all need support and understanding to know what to do with these feelings. It's not uncommon to substitute drugs, alcohol, sexual relationships, television, computers or work to mask feelings rather than understand the feelings and use them to grow.

Use the following list of resources to give you some ideas and further your understanding of what makes you feel full and fulfilled.

Resources

Books on Nutrition

David, Marc, *Nourishing Wisdom*, Bell Tower 1991.

Gittleman, Ann Louise, *Your Body Knows Best*, Pocket Books 1996.

Tribole, Evelyn and Elyse Resch, *Intuitive Eating*, St. Martins Press 1996.

Waterhouse, MS, RD, Debra, *Why Women Need Chocolate*, Hyperion 1995.

Books on Developing Intuition

Ban Breathnach, Sara, *Simple Abundance*, Warner Books 1995.

Cameron, Julia, *The Artist's Way*, G.P. Putnam & Sons 1992.

Moore, Thomas, *Care of the Soul*, Harper Collins 1992.

Myss, Caroline, *Anatomy of the Spirit*, Crown 1996.

Roth, Geneen, *Appetites: On the Search for True Nourishment*, Penguin 1997

Support Groups or Programs

Breaking Free Workshops by Geneen Roth
(Call 317-329-8445 for information.)

Over-Eaters Anonymous

Co-dependents Anonymous

Alcoholics Anonymous

Alanon

Sex and Love Addicts Anonymous

Debtors Anonymous

Narcotics Anonymous

Check your local paper or community bulletins for support groups.

Professionals

- Nutritionists *
    - Registered dietitians. Call the American Dietetic Association (800–877–1600) for a listing of dietitians in your area who specialize in working with individuals.
    - Macrobiotic nutritionists
    - Ayurvedic doctors
    - Naturopathic doctors
- Psychologists, social workers, counselors, therapists
- Exercise physiologists. (Should be certified.)
- Dance teachers
- Massage therapists
- Nurse practitioners
- Art therapists
- Music Therapists
- Spiritual directors, priests, ministers

Other:

- Creative writing and poetry classes
- Art/painting/sculpture classes
- Cooking classes
- Natural food stores
- Nature groups

* Many of these people will only be able to give you information about their best estimate of your physiological needs. We highly recommend reading Marc David's comments about this in *Nourishing Wisdom*. See reference on page 136.

chapter

24

Trusting Your Self-knowing

Just because you've now tuned in to your intuitive eater doesn't mean you should avoid any exposure to new research—or discount it. Instead, recognize that you now have a connection with your intuitive eater which has many tools at its disposal with which to filter any and all nutrition information you're exposed to. While we have presented information that we know about at the time of this writing, there will be lots more nutrition information forthcoming as nutrition research continues to shed more light on the phenomenon of why we eat the way we do or respond the way we do to what we eat. It's important for you to pay attention and expose yourself to new nutrition information. This new information will help you focus even more clearly and more rapidly to unlock the mystery of how food and your body, mind and emotions interact; you'll be able to zero in on a solution or an understanding of certain things you experience more quickly.

The activities in this book are good examples of ways your intuitive eater can filter through facts and currently available information to discover your needs. In this book, you have read about how foods may act in the human body, you experimented with these ideas, listened to how your intuitive eater responded and then, based on its signals, decided what was a good match for you and what wasn't. We encourage you to continue using this approach to explore any new information about food and/or body chemistry you come across.

And, don't limit yourself to just one nutrition resource. Explore. Play. There may be a variety of nutritionists in your town, each with a different approach—Chinese medicine, Ayurvedic, spiritual, traditional, western medical approach—some highly credentialed and others without any formal credentials who are self-trained. You may want to visit some of these. Watch newspapers and magazines for nutrition information you may want to experiment with.

Just remember, your intuitive eater is the **only** expert about your eating. Simply because an "expert" says *"This is the way,"* doesn't make it right for you. Expect to doubt yourself as you are exposed to other ideas but keep coming back to your intuitive eater as the ultimate authority.

Nutrition specialists probably *do* know more about the information they are teaching you—you have never been exposed to it before. But, they **don't** know more than you about whether their information or approach is a good match for your body. Only you can determine that. Trust yourself and your intuitive eater. There's no better way to feel full and fulfilled.

Discovering What's Right For You

1   Review your notes from the exploring you've done throughout each chapter. List at least one awareness that you were missing when you started this book which you are practicing using now.

List an awareness that you now have that you didn't have before:

_____

_____

_____

_____

_____

_____

_____

_____

_____

_____

_____

2   We suggest you periodically reread and rework the exercises in this book. Each time, you will find more ways your intuitive eater is working with you to feel full and fulfilled.

Appendix 1

U.S. Exchange System

Starch/Bread List

15 g carbohydrate, 3 g protein, trace fat, 80 calories

Amount   **Food**

Cereals/Grains/Pasta/Bread

Amount	Food
1/2 c	Bran cereals, concentrated*
1/2 c	Bran cereals, flaked*
1/2 c	Bulgar, cooked
1/2 c	Cooked cereals
2 1/2 tbs	Cornmeal, dry
3 tbs	Grapenuts
1/2 c	Grits, cooked
3/4 c	Other ready-to-eat unsweetened cereals
1/2 c	Pasta, cooked
1 1/2 c	Puffed cereals
1/3 c	Rice, white or brown, cooked
1/2 c	Shredded wheat
3 tbs	Wheat germ*

Dried Beans/Peas Lentils

Amount	Food
1/4 c	Baked beans*
1/3 c	Beans and peas, cooked, e.g. kidney, white, split, black-eyed*
1/3 c	Lentils, cooked*

Starchy Vegetables

Amount	Food
1/2 c	Corn*
1 cob	Corn on the cob, 6" long*
1/2 c	Lima beans*
1/2 c	Peas, green, canned or frozen*
1/2 c	Plantains*
1 small (3 oz)	Potato, baked
1/2 c	Potatoes, mashed
3/4 c	Squash,winter (acorn, butternut)
1/3 c	Yams, sweet potatoes, plain

Bread

1/2 (1 oz.)	Bagel
2 (2/3 oz.)	Bread sticks, crisp, 4"x1/2"
2/3 oz.	Croutons, low-fat
1/2	English muffin
1/2 (1 oz.)	Hot dog/hamburger bun
1/2 loaf	Pita, 6" across
1 (1 oz.)	Plain roll, small
1 slice (1 oz.)	Rye, pumpernickel*
1	Tortilla, 6" across
1 slice (1 oz.)	White (incl. French, Italian)
1 slice (1 oz.)	Whole Wheat

Crackers/Snacks

8	Animal crackers
3	Graham crackers, 2 1/2" sq.
3/4 oz.	Matzoh
5 slices	Melba toast
24	Oyster crackers
3 c	Popcorn, popped, no fat added
3/4 oz.	Pretzels
4	Rye crisp, 2"x3 1/2"
6	Saltine-type crackers
2 to 4 (3/4 oz.)	Whole-wheat crackers, no fat added (crisp breads)

Starch Foods Prepared with Fat
(Count as 1 starch/bread serving, plus 1 fat serving)

1	Biscuit, 2 1/2" across
1/2 c	Chow mein noodles
1 (2 oz.)	Cornbread, 2" cube
6	Crackers, round butter-type
10 (1 1/2 oz.)	French fries, 2" to 3 1/2" long
1	Muffin, plain, small
2	Pancakes, 4" across
1/4 c	Stuffing, bread, prepared
2	Taco shells, 6" across
1	Waffle, 4½" square
4 to 6 (1 oz)	Whole-wheat crackers, fat added

* 3 grams or more dietary fiber per serving. Average fiber contents of whole-grain products is 2 grams per serving. For starch foods not on this list, the general rule is that 1/2 cup cooked cereal, grain, or pasta is 1 serving: 1 ounce of a bread product is 1 serving.

Vegetable List

5 g carbohydrate, 2 g protein, 25 calories

All portion sizes, except as otherwise noted, are:
1/2 c of any cooked vegetable or vegetable juice,
1 c of any raw vegetable

Artichokes, 1/2 medium	Mushrooms
Asparagus	Okra
Bean sprouts	Onions
Beans (green, wax, Italian)	Pea pods
Beets	Rutabagas
Broccoli	Sauerkraut*
Burssel sprouts	Spinach
Cabbage	Summer squash (crookneck)
Carrots	Tomatoes, 1 large
Cauliflower	Tomato/vegetable juice*
Eggplant	Turnips
Green peppers	Water chestnuts
Greens	Zucchini
(collard, mustard, turnip)	
Kohlrabi	
Leeks	

Starchy vegetables such as corn, peas, and potatoes are found on the Starch/Bread List.

* 400 milligrams or more sodium per serving.
  Most vegetable servings contain 2 to 3 grams dietary fiber.

Meat/Meat Alternate Lists
(Protein-rich Foods)

Lean meat = 7 g protein, 3 g fat, 55 calories;
Medium-fat meat = 7 g protein, 5 g fat, 75 calories;
High-fat meat = 7 g protein, 8 g fat, 100 calories

Category	Amount	Food

Lean Meat and Alternates

Beef	1 oz	USDA Good or Choice grades of lean beef, such as round, sirloin, and flank steak; tenderloin; chipped beef
Pork	1 oz	Lean pork, such as fresh ham; canned, cured, or boiled ham; Canadian bacon; tenderloin
Veal	1 oz	All cuts are lean except veal cutlets (ground or cubed); examples of lean veal: chops and roasts
Poultry	1 oz	Chicken, turkey, Cornish hen (without skin)
Fish	1 oz	All fresh and frozen fish
	2 oz	Crab, lobster, scallops, shrimp, clams (fresh or canned in water)
	6 med.	Oysters
	1/4 c	Tuna, canned in water
	1 oz	Herring, uncreamed or smoked
	2 med.	Sardines, canned
Wild game	1 oz	Venison, rabbit, squirrel
	1 oz	Pheasant, duck, goose (no skin)
Cheese	1/4 c	Any cottage cheese
	2 tbs	Grated Parmesan
	1 oz	Diet cheeses (with less than 55 calories/oz)
Other	1 oz	95% fat-free lunch meats
	3 whites	Egg whites
	1/4 c	Egg substitutes

Medium-Fat Meat and Alternates

Beef	1 oz	Most beef products fall into this category; examples: all ground beef, roasts (rib, chuck, rump), steak (cubed, porterhouse, T-bone), meatloaf
Pork	1 oz	Most pork products fall into this category; examples: chops, loin roast, Boston butt, cutlets
Lamb	1 oz	Most lamb products fall into this category; examples: chops, leg, roast
Veal	1 oz	Cutlet, ground or cubed, unbreaded
Poultry	1 oz	Chicken (with skin), domestic duck or goose (well-drained of fat), ground turkey
Fish	1/4 c	Tuna, canned in oil and drained
	1/4 c	Salmon, canned
Cheese		Skim or part-skim milk cheese, such as:
	1/4 c	Ricotta
	1 oz	Mozzarella
	1 oz	diet cheeses (with 56 to 80 calories/oz)
Other	1 oz	85% fat-free lunch meat
	1	Egg
	4 oz	Tofu, 2½" x 2¾" x 1"
	1 oz.	Liver, hearts, kidneys, sweetbreads (high in cholesterol)

High-Fat Meat and Alternates

Beef	1 oz	Most USDA Prime cuts of beef, e.g. ribs, corned beef
Pork	1 oz.	Spareribs, ground pork, pork sausages (patties or links)
Lamb	1 oz	Patties, ground lamb
Fish	1 oz	Any fried fish product
Cheese	1 oz	All regular cheeses, e.g. American, Bleu, Cheddar, Monterey, Swiss
Other	1 oz	Lunch meats, such as bologna, salami, pimento loaf
	1 oz	Sausage, such as Polish, Italian
	1 oz	Knockwurst, smoked
	1 oz	Bratwurst
	1 (10/lb)	Frankfurters (turkey or chicken)
	1 tbs	Peanut butter (contains unsaturated fat)

Count as 1 high-fat meat plus 1 fat exchange:

1 frank	(10/lb)	Frankfurters (beef, pork, or combination)

Fruit List

15 g carbohydrate, 60 calories

All portion sizes, unless otherwise noted, are:
1/2 c fresh fruit or fruit juice, 1/4 c dried fruit.

Amount   **Food**

Fresh, Frozen, and Unsweetened Canned Fruit

Amount	Food
1	Apple, raw, 2" across
1/2 c	Applesauce, unsweetened
4	Apricots, medium, raw
1/2 c (4 halves)	Apricots, canned
1/2	Banana, 9" long
3/4 c	Blackberries, raw*
3/4 c	Blueberries, raw*
1/3	Cantaloupe, 5" across
1 c	Cantaloupe, cubes
12	Cherries, large, raw
1/2 c	Cherries, canned
2	Figs, raw, 2" across
1/2 c	Fruit cocktail, canned
1/2	Grapefruit, medium
3/4 c	Grapefruit, segments
15	Grapes, small
1/8	Honeydew melon, medium
1 c	Honeydew melon, cubes
1	Kiwi, large
3/4 c	Mandarin oranges
1/2	Mango, small
1	Nectarine, 1½" across
1	Orange, 2½" across
1 c	Papaya
1 (3/4 c)	Peach, 2¾" across
1/2 c (2 halves)	Peaches, canned
1/2 large or 1 small	Pear
1/2 c (2 halves)	Pears, canned
2	Persimmons, medium, native
3/4 c	Pineapple, raw
1/3 c	Pineapple, canned

2	Plums, raw, 2" across
1/2	Pomegranate*
1 c	Raspberries, raw*
1 1/4 c	Strawberries, raw, whole*
2	Tangerines, 2½" across
1 1/4 c	Watermelon, cubes

Dried Fruit

4 rings	Apples*
7 halves	Apricots*
2 1/2 medium	Dates
1 1/2	Figs*
3 medium	Prunes*
2 tbs	Raisins

Fruit Juice

1/2 c	Apple juice/cider
1/3 c	Cranberry Juice cocktail
1/3 c	Grape juice
1/2 c	Grapefruit juice
1/2 c	Orange juice
1/2 c	Pineapple juice
1/3 c	Prune juice

* 3 grams or more dietary fiber per serving.
Average fiber contents of fresh, frozen, and dry fruits:
2 grams per serving.

Milk List
(Protein-rich Foods)

Nonfat and very low-fat milk =
12 g carbohydrate, 8 g protein, trace fat, 90 calories
Low-fat milk =
12 g carbohydrate, 8 g protein, 5 g fat, 120 calories
Whole milk =
12 g carbohydrate, 8 g protein, 8 g fat, 150 calories

Amount	Food
Nonfat and Very Low-Fat Milk	
1 c	Nonfat milk
1 c	½% milk
1 c	1% milk
1/3 c	Dry nonfat milk
1/2 c	Evaporated nonfat milk
1 c	Low-fat buttermilk
8 oz	Plain nonfat yogurt
1/4 c	Fat-free cream cheese
Low-Fat Milk	
1 c fluid	2% milk
8 oz	Plain low-fat yogurt, with added nonfat milk solids
Whole Milk	
1 c	Whole milk
1/2 c	Evaporated whole milk
8 oz	Whole plain yogurt

Fat List

5 g fat, 45 calories

Amount   **Food**

Unsaturated Fats

Amount	Food
1/8 medium	Avocados
1 tsp	Margarine
1 tbs	Margarine, diet
1 tsp	Mayonnaise
1 tbs	Mayonnaise, reduce calorie
	Nuts and seeds:
6 whole	Almonds, dry roasted
1 tbs	Cashews, dry roasted
20 small or 10 large	Peanuts
2 whole	Pecans
2 tsp	Pumpkin seeds
1 tbs	Other nuts
1 tbs	Seeds, pine nuts, sunflower seeds (without shells)
2 whole	Walnuts
1 tsp	Oil (corn, cottonseed, safflower, soybean, sunflower, olive, peanut)
10 small or 5 large	Olives
1 tbs	Salad dressing, all varieties
2 tsp	Salad dressing, mayonnaise type
1 tbs	Salad dressing, mayonnaise type, reduced calorie
2 tbs	Salad dressing, reduced calorie

Saturated Fats

1 slice	Bacon
1 tsp	Butter
1/2 oz.	Chitterlings
2 tbs	Coconut, shredded
2 tbs	Coffee whitener, liquid
4 tsp	Coffee whitener, powder
1 tbs	Cream (heavy, whipping)
2 tbs	Cream (light, coffee, table)
2 tbs	Cream (sour)
1 tbs	Cream cheese
1/4 oz.	Salt pork

Appendix 2

Quick Meal Ideas

Each meal listed contains foods supplying protein, carbohydrates, and fats. Each food is labeled with a **P** for protein, **C** for carbohydrate, and **F** for fat.

Using your experiences from the *"Discovering What's Right For You"* sections in each chapter, you will want to alter the serving sizes of each food to make sure you are satisfied and not eating too little or too much. You will need different quantities at different times depending on your own intuitive eater's signals. And, if you found that your body feels better with high protein meals, then you will want to have a larger serving of those items labeled **P** for protein and choose smaller servings of the foods labeled **C** and/or delete some of the **C** foods planned. Appendix 1 lists foods rich in carbohydrate or protein and an average serving size. These are not given to tell you the size serving to eat. Your intuitive eater will tell you that. Instead, these are provided to help you compose a meal that varies in proportion of protein to carbohydrate. A high protein meal is usually at least 2 proteins to 1 carbohydrate.

For example:

P Omelet (eggs scrambled with frozen cooked chopped onions, peppers, canned mushrooms)
Top omelet with: salsa
  F olives
  F low fat sour cream
C Oven fries (cut a potato and/or yam into strips. Spray with non-stick spray. Bake at 500° for 15–20 minutes or until brown)
C Fresh fruit salad

If you need a high protein meal, you could:

♦   choose to delete either the fries or the fruit

♦   choose small servings of both fries and fruit in comparison to
     your servings of eggs

♦   choose to prepare a larger number of eggs and have regular
     portions of fries and fruit

Quick Meals

Fresh Pasta (grocery deli)
C   Fresh pasta
      Microwave vegetables (fresh produce section)
      or frozen vegetables (polybag)
      Bottled Marinara sauce
P   Chicken fillets cut into strips and microwaved or
      boneless skinless breast or fresh or frozen shrimp
C   Italian bread
P,F Parmesan cheese
C   Fresh, cored pineapple
C   Arrowroot cookies or graham crackers

Tossed Salad
      Tossed salad from produce section of grocery store.
P   Lean deli meat
F   Bottled low fat salad dressing (or salad dressing mix &
      equal amounts buttermilk and low-fat mayo)
C   Croutons, whole grain bread or crackers

Soup Dinner
      Broth based vegetable soup (canned or packet,
      may have chicken/beef in it)
      Add fresh or plain, frozen vegetables
C   Add cooked brown rice, cracked wheat,
      drained can of beans, peas, corn, potatoes
P   Lean, chopped chicken, ham deli meats, tofu
      Tomatoes—canned dehydrated minced onion and
      garlic, fresh or dried herbs
C,F Cornbread from mix
P,F Packaged grated cheese to top cornbread or soup

Baked Potato Dinner
C   Baked potato (microwaved)
P,F Low-fat sour cream, yogurt
P   Chopped lean meats or low-fat cottage cheese
      Cooked vegetables (fresh or plain, frozen),
      (steamed/microwaved)

Frozen Dinner, Plus
(Most low-fat frozen dinners have 2 Ps and 1 C. Typically, people would need two low-fat frozen dinners to get a high protein meal.)
P   Tyson chicken dinner, Weight Watchers, Lean Cuisine, Budget Gourmet, or Benihana Lights
        vegetables, steamed or microwaved
C   Whole grain bread or steamed brown/wild rice or baked potato
F   Butter or dressing to top vegetables, potato, or bread

Cheese Toast/Fruit Salad or Vegetable Salad
C,P Whole wheat bread with mustard and cottage cheese, Canadian bacon, or low-fat cheese, broiled
C   Fruit salad—any or all or the following: strawberries, pineapple, banana, blueberries.
        Sprinkle with a few nuts (**F**), raisins (**C**), dry cereals (**C**).

        Vegetable salad—toss lettuce and spinach with cherry tomatoes and sprouts
F   Add a low fat dressing.

Muffin/Fruit Salad/Cheese
C   Whole Grain muffin or English Muffin
C   Fruit salad, as above
P,F Cheese (feta, cheddar, cottage) in or beside salad

Pizza/Vegetable Salad
C   Lavosh crackers or pita or English muffin or rice cakes or package of prepared pizza crust topped with the following:
P   Lean ground beef
P,F Low-fat cheese (mozzarella, jack, farmers, feta)
        Pizza sauce, oregano, parsley, basil, onion or garlic powder
        Bell peppers and onions (chopped frozen or fresh), mushrooms (fresh or canned)
        Broil until cheese melts.
        Vegetable salad, as above; toss with Italian spices and Parmesan (**P, F**)

Grilled Patties/Vegetables/Salad/Bread or Grain
P   Mix canned tuna, salmon, or chicken with an egg and seasonings (onion, parsley, etc,) and grill in a non-stick pan

C,F   Gravy/sauce from seasoning packets to top the patties
Broccoli (squash, tomato, steamed cabbage with caraway, cauliflower). Look in healthy-food cookbooks for more ideas for vegetables

C   Whole grain bread, brown rice, noodles

Shrimp Creole/Salad/Bread
P   Shrimp (frozen or fresh), heated with tomatoes and tomato sauce, steamed celery, onions, peppers, okra, creole spices.

C   Instant rice
Lettuce tossed with raw vegetables

F   Salad dressing

C   Sourdough bread

Omelette/Toast/Vegetable/Fruit
P   Eggs scrambled in a non-stick pan with frozen, cooked, chopped onions and peppers, mushrooms (canned or cooked). Add chopped tomatoes or salsa, a dab of sour cream (**F**).

C   Whole wheat toast or "Oven Fries." (Cut a baked potato into strips and season lightly with oil and bake for 30 minutes.)

C   Fruit salad

Steak/Potato/Vegetable/Salad
P,F   Broiled filet or (marinated round or flank steak, chicken breast, fish steak or filet)

C   Boiled or baked potato; rice, plain or with raisins and nuts
Green beans and mushrooms, microwaved

F   Tossed salad and low-fat dressing

Steamed Vegetables/Rice/Cheese

      Vegetable medley (fresh, packaged, ready-to-cook or frozen)

C   Try adding fruit like pineapple or apples or raisins to the vegetables (particularly if they are bell peppers, cabbage and onion)

C   Instant brown rice

P,F   Packaged grated cheese on top. Top cooked rice with cooked vegetables mixed with fruits.
      Top with grated cheese.

Taco Salad/Fruit

      Lettuce, chili peppers, chili powder, salsa

P   Lean ground beef or chicken cooked in powdered taco seasoning (from a packet)

P,F   Grated cheese

C   Canned pinto or kidney beans

C   Tortilla chips broken into salad

C   Strawberries, fresh or frozen or other unsweetened fruit

Burrito/Fruit

C   Whole wheat flour tortilla filled with items below.

C   Pinto, kidney beans, drained or refried beans

P,F   Low-fat cheese in tortilla
      drained, canned zucchini, canned carrots, canned tomatoes, bake at 350 for 10 minutes
      Lettuce, tomato or salsa on side or top

C   Fresh orange or other fresh or frozen fruit

Quesadilla/fruit

C   Whole wheat flour tortilla
      Fresh spinach, sliced fresh mushrooms

P,F   Shredded low-fat cheese
      fold in half, microwave

C   Add fresh fruit or fruit salad

Chinese Stir Fry

P   Chicken, boneless skinless, cut in strips, or
        lean round steak, cut across grain in thin strips, or
        tofu. Cook in large skillet treated with nonstick
        spray or a little oil. Add couple of tablespoons of
        water to keep it from sticking. Then add frozen
        green peppers, carrots, mushrooms, broccoli,
        onions, snow peas, canned water chestnuts, canned
        bamboo shoots, soy sauce, garlic powder, onion
        powder, ground ginger, a little pineapple juice
C   Instant brown rice
C   Orange sections

Pasta Salad

C   Boil whole grain pasta shells, curls, elbows, etc.
        until just soft. Drain, rinse with cold water.
        Add broccoli, cauliflower, tomatoes, carrots,
        green peppers and
F   Low-fat Italian dressing.
        Refrigerate.
P   Add farmers cheese or lean turkey, chicken, tuna.
C   Fruit

Chicken Parmesan

P   Boneless chicken breast without skin.
        Cook until half done in microwave or in skillet
        treated with nonstick spray on stove.
P,F   Cover with low-fat mozzarella and spaghetti sauce
        from jar. Sprinkle lightly with Parmesan cheese.
        Microwave or bake.
C   Spinach salad with mushrooms, reduced calorie
        Italian dressing, whole wheat noodles.
C   Bread

Hot Cereal

C   Hot cereal: oatmeal, Kashi, or Cream of Wheat, etc.
P   Cook using milk to replace the water required.
        Add dry, powdered milk if you need even more
        protein with the cereal.
C   Fruit, fresh or dried

Chili
P   Tofu or TVP (textured vegetable protein),
       ground beef, turkey, or stew beef.
       Tomatoes, frozen chopped green and red peppers,
       onions
C   Canned, drained beans—black beans, kidney beans,
       garbanzo beans
C,F   Cornbread (from mix)
F   Tossed salad/dressing

Index

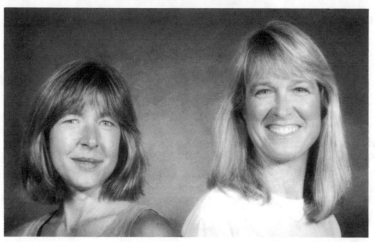

Photo: Leila Grossman

Nan Allison, MS, RD is a licensed nutritionist, and co-owner of Allison and Beck Nutrition Consultants, Inc., Nashville's premier nutrition firm since its inception in 1987.

Her ongoing interest in why individuals and cultures choose to eat the way they do led her to specialize in working with people who have spent their lives struggling with food and weight.

A native Tennessean who spent most of her childhood in India, Nan earned her bachelors degree with high honors from the University of Tennessee, and her masters degree in nutrition science from Tufts University. She completed her dietetic internship at Frances Stern Nutrition Center of New England Medical Center Hospital.

Her career in nutrition has spanned two continents—from refugee camps in Thailand, consulting and lecturing in Japan, to developing nutrition education programs for businesses, and for the federal Women, Infants, and Children (WIC) Program in Tennessee. She developed nutrition curriculum and taught extensively at three universities in Nashville, and served as assistant professor of nutrition at Meharry Medical College.

Carol Beck, MS is a nutrition therapist, artist, author and co-owner of Allison and Beck Nutrition Consultants. Carol specializes in working with the most difficult eating-disorder and weight-loss/gain cases or the "non-compliant patient." Ninety-eight percent of her clients are referrals from psychotherapists, physicians, other nutritionists, clients, and treatment centers. On a daily basis, she guides people through their journeys toward intuitive eating. Carol is creating another set of books entitled **Colors of Loss,** a collection of watercolors and poetry about grief and loss. She also writes a regular column for *Daughters* newsletter.

A native Californian, she earned her bachelor's degree, with honors, in dietetics from the University of California, and her master's degree in health education from the University of North Texas. She completed her dietetic internship at Presbyterian Medical Center in Dallas, Texas.

Carol has spent her professional life writing and speaking about nutrition and health. Her work experience includes seven years conducting programs and writing nutrition education materials as nutrition education coordinator at University of North Texas. In addition, she served as an instructor in nutrition.

Upon moving to Tennessee, Carol served as assistant professor at Tennessee State University. Her responsibilities included writing and designing more than 20 nutrition publications, one of which won the Cavender Award for Outstanding Publication and the International Association of Business Communicators Excellence Award. She has traveled throughout the region presenting some 500 programs and workshops for both the public and for health professionals.

How many others do you know who might benefit from the ideas and information to be found in *Full and Fulfilled?* Show someone you care. It's a gift to be treasured and appreciated.

If you're unable to find additional copies of *Full and Fulfilled* at your local book or natural food store, use the order form below.

Please send _____ copies of *Full and Fulfilled* to:

Name _____

Phone (_____) _____

Address _____

City _____ State _____ Zip _____

Enclose a check made payable to A&B Books for $16.95 per book (includes shipping, handling, and sales tax). Mail to:

A&B Books
2826 Azalea Place
Nashville, TN 37204

To pay by credit card,
call 800/345-6665.